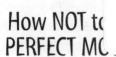

How NOT to
PERFECT MOTHER

Libby Purves is a novelist, journalist and broadcaster.
She lives in Suffolk with her husband Paul Heiney
and their student son and daughter.

Also by Libby Purves

Britain at Play
How Not to Raise a Perfect Child
The Sailing Weekend Book (with Paul Heiney)
One Summer's Grace
How Not to Be a Perfect Family

How NOT to Be a PERFECT MOTHER

The crafty mother's guide to a quiet life

Libby Purves

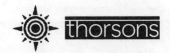

Thorsons
An Imprint of HarperCollins*Publishers*
77–85 Fulham Palace Road,
Hammersmith, London W6 8JB

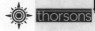

and *Thorsons* are trademarks of
HarperCollins*Publishers* Ltd

The website address is: www.thorsonselement.com

First published in paperback by Fontana 1986
First published in paperback by Thorsons 1994
This edition published 2004

10 9 8 7 6 5 4 3 2 1

© Libby Purves 2004

Libby Purves asserts the moral right to
be identified as the author of this work

A catalogue record of this book
is available from the British Library

ISBN 0 00 716384 3

All illustrations by Viv Quillin

Printed and bound in Great Britain by
Clays Ltd, St Ives Plc, Bungay

Contents

To my children, and Paul

Acknowledgements

Grateful thanks for advice and example to:

Joyce and Virginia Ash
Janet Bellis
Clare Brindley
Judy Brooks
Anna Carragher
Tina Clubb
Belinda Devenish
Helen Fraser
Jill Freud
Nikki Freud
Sarah Gleadell
Valerie Grove
Sandy Guertin
Fiona Hamilton
Lynn Hurst
Wendy Jobson
Priscilla Lamont
Wiz Mosson
Tina Potter
Lorraine Price

Judy Purves
Debbie Pyn
Natasha Quested
Jenny Rogers
Anna Southall
Penny Steel
Sheridan Steen
Caroline Stevens
Heather Taylor
Lynn Templeton
Valentine Thornhill
Teresa Walsh
Nicky Wilson
Sally Wright

… and many others

And, of course, my mother

Libby Purves, 2004

Preface, 2004

I wrote this book because 20 years ago I needed to read it, and it wasn't there. Contemplating my new son in his hospital cot, or struggling with his wakefulness during long, long nights, I wanted a book that acknowledged that I had feelings, too. I wanted someone to admit that perfection in motherhood is impossible, that not everything can be planned or scheduled, and that to get through the day with an infant all you need is love – which comes pretty easily to most of us – commonsense, good-humour and a great deal of rat-like cunning.

There were a lot of perfectionist baby-books around at the time, focused (understandably) on the needs of the child and frankly rather careless about the parents in charge. So, during the turbulent years while I had two children under three, I made notes. When I began writing, with the youngest in a basket under the table and the eldest rampaging round on a plastic Thomas the Tank Engine which took lumps of plaster off the kitchen wall, I was still in the thick of it, on the front line, hunched over a typewriter at the kitchen table. But I knew that I didn't know it all, because we all lead different lives in different styles. So I began by circulating a rather tatty questionnaire round 50 mothers I knew. They were of different ages, types, incomes and generations, but all of them were women who seemed to me to be doing, or to have done in the past, a pretty good job of it.

I just asked how they handled the daily round – bath-time, tantrums, feeding, dressing, sleep, biting, the lot. Their answers were magnificently diverse, cheerful, fond, resigned and occasionally a bit bizarre. They encouraged me greatly. So I wrote this book, and launched it off into the world in the hope of sharing that encouragement and pleasure with other mothers. To my amazement it has never been out of print since, and has been translated into a dozen languages. Babies, clearly, are an international language. They do not change with passing fashions.

However, the century has turned and now the time seems ripe to examine and revise *How Not to Be a Perfect Mother*. Above all, baby equipment has changed: there were points that needed updating (when did you last see a carrycot?). In some ways the attitude to mothers has changed as well. In the early 1980s a baby was not yet the designer accessory it has become since. Film stars did not push buggies around where cameras might see them. Now that Rachel-from-*Friends* and Miranda-from-*Sex-in-the-City* brandish babies in fiction, and Madonna Ritchie and Catherine Zeta Jones are photographed toting infants with all the carefree style of pashminas or Prada bags, there is a new and different pressure. You may fall for the danger-ous illusion that it is possible not only to be a perfect loving mother – and probably a worker too, for some of the time – but to remain chic and *soignée* as well, fit for a *Hello!* magazine spread. And that is just as much nonsense as the old idea that a grown-up busy working girl would mutate into a calm, milky household angel by the mere fact of giving birth.

Contemplating all this, it seemed a good moment to revise the book a little. I have not changed much, except a few tenses and some advice on modern equipment, because the essence of the original *How Not to Be a Perfect Mother* was that it came straight from the coalface of practical early motherhood. There is nothing more irritating to the new mother than being given sanctimonious advice by some middle-aged woman who gets enough sleep and whose children are big enough to be sent up ladders to fix bits of loose guttering. So I have tried to leave intact the original tone of the book, even when it verges on the mildly hysterical.

But I would also like to take the opportunity to say that the friendships and contacts I made in the years after this book was published have – however brief and fleeting some of them were – meant a great deal to me. This book has become, across ages and backgrounds and some national borders, a kind of club. We look one another in the eye – having met perhaps in some quite different context – and both say, 'Yup. That's how it was. That's how it is, and always will be.' The extraordinary, taxing, inspiring, despairing, exhausting and energizing experience of having a baby and caring for it through the infant years is something no mother ever forgets. And not many fathers, either. To all who went through it alongside me, and have shared the experience since and nodded in recognition of the way this book told it, I am happy to dedicate this new edition, with real love. And, as we say these days, respect!

Introduction

A mother's duty is quite clear: it is to be perfect. Mothers, as we all know, are sacred. They are sweet, loving, caring, self-denying madonnas. They are always there. They have tender bosoms and endless patience. A mother is like the legendary pelican, ripping her own breast to feed her young. Any mother would lay down her life for her child ...

Well, yes, true enough. I am a mother, and *I would* lay down my life for my children; but I see no reason to do it every single day. Under the mantle of every mother lies an ordinary, disgruntled human being: there is no special saint-factory churning out tranquil and self-sacrificing madonnas. Every carefree, adventurous, selfish girl-in-the-street is at risk of being conscripted to wear a mother's halo. And the transition from healthy adult selfishness to

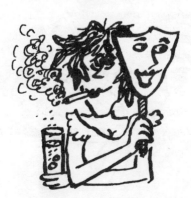

the status of maternal angel can be a painful one: rather like a butterfly trying to climb back into the chrysalis. It is that transition, in the early years, which is the subject of this book.

Nature helps the process along: in the first days, the urge to perfect pelicanhood is strong. When a baby is born, the average woman becomes chronically unselfish. The infant lies there in a plastic hospital cot, hypnotizing her with its beady blue eyes; and although she hurts all over and her head is still spinning, her baby's willpower can bend her exhaustion to its demands. It sucks busily, works out its own sleeping schedule with reference to nobody, wets its nappy whenever it feels like it, and feeds eccentrically – three times an hour and then not for ages. Place any small obstacle in the path of the baby's inexorable will and it will scream at a pitch carefully programmed to exact immediate maternal obedience. It demands conversation at midnight but falls rudely asleep in the middle of

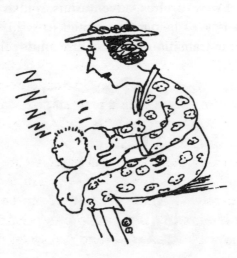

Granny's best nursery rhyme; a baby has no manners, no consideration, and no responsibilities. It just gets on with growing bigger.

Confronted by this tyrant, you drop everything and swim with the tide, serving the baby and forgetting that you ever had preferences of your own. At first, this makes good sense; for a few months after a birth, nobody should expect much beyond survival and the odd quiet drink in front of the television. The problem is that the habit of self-obliteration tends to carry on for too long, reinforced by the sentimental picture we have of motherhood. Sometimes, the reasonable doctrine of 'demand feeding' continues unreasonably for 18 years, and widens to embrace demand washing-up of teenage midnight feasts and demand lending of the family car every Saturday night. Even in the early days, we overdo the sacrifice: we leave the house on freezing days with the children wrapped like Eskimos, but too preoccupied to put on our own coats. We stop every conversation five times a minute to wipe noses and respond to insistent little voices at knee-level; we walk miles in blizzards to buy finger-paints (well, I did, once). After a few years of this, we end up dressed like bag ladies and apologizing to everybody. For the most extremely unselfish mothers, the ones with no pleasures of their own, are often the ones who feel most guilty and depressed.

There is enormous pleasure in being a parent. It is fun to watch a baby grow, and smile and talk and begin to invent mad private games with bits of old hosepipe and buckets of sand; but it is also cripplingly hard graft. It is *inescapable* work: even professional nannies and nurses, when their own first babies are born, have been reduced to tears by the realization that now there will be no days off. A mother's working day can stretch to 18 hours or more if she lets it.

But why should we let it? If there are corners to cut, which hurt nobody, why not cut them? Why not bend the baby to your own convenience every now and then? May not a saint put her feet up with a beer and a book occasionally?

This book is about the way real, fallible mothers *really* get through the day. There are plenty of technical baby manuals on the market: some are excellent, some manage to make bathing a baby sound as complicated as stripping down a MIG fighter engine; nearly all of them are perfectionist in tone. This is an *imperfectionist* book, about the cheerful cutting of corners, without guilt.

Of course you have to look after babies and small children properly. It is hard not to, when every whimper of fright or trembling lip can strike you with agonized sympathy. But with a bit of low cunning, you can win a part of your own life back, and do the child no harm. Squaddies in the army have always understood this principle: the war has to be fought, and possibly your life sacrificed, but in the process you can work the system, sneak the extra chocolate into your knapsack, and get a kip behind the cookhouse while someone else peels your load of potatoes. You stop short of treason or desertion, but there are always rules to bend.

From madonna-and-child to Sergeant Bilko is a bit of a comedown for your image, perhaps; but it is much easier to live up to, and considerably more fun. Sometimes, as

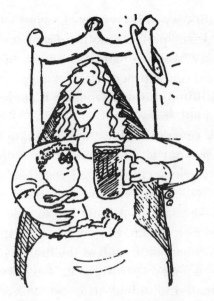

Bilko, you actually do the same things that the perfection-ists would have you do, but for slightly different reasons. During the worst difficulties of early breastfeeding, when no theoretical benefit to the baby compensates for the pain, I kept myself going on the thought that the more breast milk I got down the baby, the less chance there was of having to nurse him through frightening baby illnesses. Or take discipline: I once watched two mothers at tea, both pestered by their toddlers. One kept saying: 'Don't touch the mug, darling, it's hot, it might burn you.' The other mother put it differently: 'Don't touch that mug, darling. It's *Mummy's*.' I noticed that the latter one managed to drink her tea, fending the little beast off with her arm and defending her rights; whereas the former put her mug up on a nice safe shelf and never touched a drop. She left, tired and thirsty, for another gruelling bathtime of creative water-play and coaxing. I suspect that the more selfish and least 'perfect' mother (who, no doubt, used bathtime as a chance to paint her own toenails while the child splashed undisturbed) was the happier woman. And as for the children, I doubt whether it made much difference to them either way.

This book covers the first three years, or a little more, depending on your child. I have never seen the point of lumping 'preschool children' all together; it is the first three years which contain the maximum bewilderment and the fastest changes. A baby has landed, as alien as a UFO, as odd as a dream. Slowly he turns into something more like a human adult, and as the fourth year begins, he has travelled a long way towards it. You have, at three and a half, a small individual who can talk enough to be reasoned with, who knows (although he may not agree) that fair is fair and orders is orders. You are not forever having to coax him to lie on his back while you change nappies; he can communicate with strangers and eat with a knife and fork.

At this age, too, children become widely different individuals. Not that they aren't individuals before three; but early on, the common qualities far outweigh the differences. *All* six-month-old babies grab the spoon when you try to feed them; *all* new walkers pull things off tables on to their heads; and the particular qualities of a two-year-old (not unlike a suitcaseful of gelignite on a bouncy castle) are pretty universal too. But after four years you may have acquired a tough gunslinger or a dainty Victorian miss (of either sex); an intellectual or an athlete or a socialite. They stand apart from one another, small but separate, each on a private platform of heredity and chance and conditioning. So a mature three seemed a good age at which to stop; it is also the period which I know best from my own life. To fill in the gaps and catch the great and ingenious variety of mothering styles, I consulted 50 friends, with 86 children between them. Some are of my generation, some older or younger; some working mothers, some housewives, some single parents. To all of them I am boundlessly grateful for their advice, confessions, encouragement and occasional reproofs.

One final apology. These days, writers have to tie themselves in knots trying to be fair to both sexes (back in the days of Truby King a baby was 'he', and that was that). Some writers say 'he/she' and 'his/hers' all the time, or else alternate 'he' and 'she' so that you get a disquieting impression of a running sex-change; some bravely confess that since theirs are all boys or all girls, they will stick to the sex they know best. Nobody dares to say 'it' any more, even of a foetus, lest the mothers should be mortally offended.

I have one of each sex, myself. And after much thought, I have decided to use *he, she* and *it* indiscriminately and according to my mood. I hope it does not annoy you too much. After all, nobody's perfect.

• •

Chapter One

Pregnant, Proud
and Panic-stricken

When I was first pregnant, and prone to describe every last flutter and twinge to everyone I met, I went to lunch with a friend who already had a couple of children under two. I sat in my circular splendour, hands folded on my vast bump, while she mopped and wiped, and caught toppling high-chairs, and embarked on wild, hopeless lines of reasoning about Teddy eating up his carrots and the discarded rabbit-slipper not wanting to sit in the milk-pan *really*. For the first time, at that moment, it occurred to me that pregnancy is a lousy sort of preparation for motherhood.

When you are pregnant, you buy new clothes, think about your diet, avoid lifting, put your feet up, and dwell endlessly on every gripe and swelling of your precious body. You attend classes about your internal organs, watch your fingers anxiously for signs of oedema, and are told to feel proud of yourself. Once the baby arrives, what happens? You never get your feet up, you live off discarded Marmite soldiers, wear old shirts covered with sicked-up banana, and have to lift a great lump of a baby around all day.

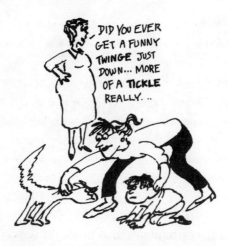

As for the precious internal organs, you would hardly notice if you got appendicitis; and nor would anyone else. All that pregnancy really prepares you for is the birth – which, however tough, is basically an event at which you are the centre of attention. People put pillows behind you, and everyone keeps saying how well you are doing ('Six centimetres dilated! Well done, Mum!'). You never think of preparing for all the years *after* these exciting few hours, when you are just the harassed rag-bag in the background to your baby and when – far from telling you how well you are doing – the world blames you squarely for every spot, bruise, tantrum and beer-can thrown off the Millwall terraces. There do exist a few classes labelled 'Education for Parenthood', but none which includes running a commando course through a maze of weaving sit-on buses, carrying a bowl of apple slime, answering mad questions, and never once taking your eye off the tense dialogue between the two-year-old and the cat.

Women who already have children, like my friend,

have little patience with the processes of other people's first pregnancies. I remember offering a magazine editor my emotionally acute 'Diary of Nine Months' and explaining how fascinating it was that while I started out by feeling vulnerable yet protective, by the third month I felt, well, sort of protective yet vulnerable; and how useful airline sick-bags were on the Underground. Editor had a child of her own, so her eyes glazed over a bit; but she gamely agreed to print this rubbish. However, by the time I got around to finishing it, my son was born and I, in turn, could not see what all the fuss had been about.

So it is with some diffidence that I offer a chapter on pregnancy and its problems. I can only say that, at the time, they seemed as enormous as I was.

The most useful side-effect of being pregnant is the Cousin Elizabeth complex (see Luke 1:39-41!). This is an overwhelming urge to visit other pregnant women and compare notes. It makes you some very good and useful friends, who you are going to need later on. And women in waiting together invariably become horribly intimate; we tell one another the most amazingly frank things about our various membranes and urges, as if preparing for the utter shamelessness of the maternity ward. (In a postnatal unit, if a TV repairman walks in wearing a white coat, half a dozen novice mothers start ripping at their clothing and trying to discuss their nipples, piles and stitches.)

Since encounters with actual mothers tend to bring on the sort of shamefaced guilt that I felt during that chaotic lunch with the two babies, other newly pregnant women are essential if you want company in which to discuss the various exciting developments under your smock. You can also share your innocent idealism about children, which for some reason seems to enrage people already toiling at the coalface of motherhood. If you plan to give birth standing up, to the sound of Mozart, or underwater with a Radical Midwife standing by with raspberry-leaf tea, you can ramble on about your 'birthing' theories to your Cousin-Elizabeth friend. If you plan to stimulate your newborn to genius with flash-cards and breastfeed for five long years, fine; tell her all about it. If you have visions of perfectly ironed flounces surrounding a delicate cradle, set in a flowery room lined with shelves of terry nappies as white and soft as swan's down, tell her about that, too; and have nice little chats about fabric-softener. Argue with your friend about nannies, about state education, the importance of surrounding the child with Art, the morality of 'Red Riding Hood'. Smile radiantly at everybody, dream your dreams; say how disgusting the title of this book is, and plan a life of serene self-sacrifice. You will be down here with the rest of us soon enough, learning mother-cunning. Welcome.

Meanwhile, there are the ailments and irritations of pregnancy itself to deal with. It is a bit like being hijacked, or having squatters in. You suddenly have an important, vulnerable, determined little passenger, curled up comfortably in there, shoving your stomach and bladder hither and yon, taking what it needs without a by-your-leave. You, for instance, will get seriously anaemic before the baby runs short of iron. As to food, healthy babies have been born to half-starved mothers. The baby is in charge. All you can do is to make sure that it isn't forced to have anything it shouldn't, like cigarette smoke, alcohol or drugs. With

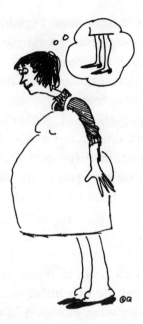

every new research document, these indulgences grow
harder and harder to countenance; no sooner has one lot of
gloomy doctors concluded that 'even one glass of wine a
day' may damage a foetus, than another lot wades in with
the conclusion that the unborn 'flinches and squirms away'
when a mother even allows the *thought* of a cigarette to
cross her mind. There are books more medical than this to
persuade you one way or the other. All I offer is my own
selfish reasoning: it kept me down to a couple of glasses of
wine a week and not even a single paracetamol for two lots
of nine months. I just used to tell myself that this baby *had*
to be born exceptionally big and strong and shockproof,
because it was going to have a less than perfect mother.
This tactic worked. Every drink turned down, every additive-
burger rejected, seemed like a form of insurance against

having a fretful, sickly baby later. I could not defend this line of reasoning in court, but it kept me perfectly happy and abstemious through two pregnancies.

Coming off the booze and cigarettes, however, is a mild problem. Other physical matters are more intrusive. (The only merciful dispensation of providence that I can remember is that just when your ankles have swollen so revoltingly that you can hardly bear to look at them, your bump shoots out so far that you can't see them anyway.) Here are a few comments and a few cures for *the ailments of pregnancy*:

Antenatal clinics

It may seem odd to list a clinic under 'ailments of pregnancy', but after a couple of routine antenatals in a big hospital, you will see why. However good a hospital is about the actual birth, the odds are that its clinic is terrible. Appointments are made in great batches, all for the same time, so that mothers (even with sad, wailing toddlers) sometimes have to wait several hours after their official time. My personal best is 2 hours 55 minutes. Even then, all that may happen is a blood test, followed by another long sit, followed by a urine test and a hop on to the scales; then another sit, and a desultory chat with a student midwife. Incidentally, it pays to learn the belts of the nurses on your first visit: students, junior and senior midwives have different colours. Do not waste your valuable time asking some 18-year-old student questions; grab someone with a belt that has been *earned*.

On my first-ever visit, I sat bursting with anxious questions while the 'booking form' was laboriously filled in by a very junior nurse indeed. She asked severely, 'Right. Now. Contact with dates? Have you had contact with dates?' Dates? Dates! My God, I thought, they're not toxic, are they? Dates don't produce abnormalities in foetuses? I remembered the panic about the green potatoes a few years before. And I had eaten stuffed dates only the week before! Oh, no! 'Contact with dates?' repeated the child, pencil poised, obviously writing me off as one of the poor dim underclass mothers they teach you about at training school. 'Well?' Recovering my balance, I snatched the form off her and read: 'GERMAN MEASLES (RUBELLA), CONTACT WITH: Dates:'. She had missed a line. These encounters do little to soothe the nervous primagravida.

When your big moment comes, you are led into a cubicle, asked to take off your lower garments, and lie on a padded plank until The Consultant comes round. Even sitting up to read your book or ease your heartburn may be treated as insubordination and Wasting Doctor's Time (what doctor? where?).

After a couple of hours of this persecution, a nervous woman will become hopelessly docile, too timid to ask questions even if they are burning in her heart; and the more spirited, bolshie type becomes so rude that she, too, forgets to ask the questions that make her cry secretly in the night.

None of this is any good. Plenty of people have campaigned to improve British antenatal cattle clinics, and they are making slow but sure progress. Rudeness, insensitivity and inattention are regularly exposed by the dutiful media. Occasionally one hospital lays itself open to ridicule or disgust, and all the others pull up their socks an inch or two. I did most especially enjoy the tale of the woman who miscarried and insisted she was still pregnant. She demanded an ultrasound scan, but was refused one. Eventually, she was admitted against her will to a mental hospital for being obsessively demented about this phantom baby. When she escaped and got her scan, it turned out she *was* still pregnant. She had only miscarried one of twins. The baby was born safely, and the hospital, according to reports, 'apologized'. Apologized! It should have been put in the stocks!

Plenty of midwives campaign to improve the system; depending on where you live, you might be luckier than someone else. Meanwhile, there are a few ways of improving your lot:

- If you live in an area where you are expected to go to the hospital for every visit, ask for 'shared care', so that half your appointments are mere visits to your own GP. If you don't like your GP, or he looks gloomy at the thought of obstetrics and new babies (some doctors positively prefer cosy chats about arthritis and golf), then for heaven's sake change your GP. Quick. A doctor who doesn't like pregnant women is not going to be overjoyed when you turn up with a new baby covered in mysterious spots, either, or when you dither for weeks over the whooping-cough jab. Change doctors! Now!
- At the hospital, make sure you always book the first appointment of the morning, and get there 20 minutes before it. Then nobody can say, 'Doctor's running a bit late this morning.'

- Take something to read. The hospital supply of mysteriously stained two-year-old copies of *OK!* magazine can seriously damage your morale.
- Alternatively, knit. Everyone knits in antenatal clinics, sometimes managing a whole sweater while waiting for God to sweep in in his white coat. Or you can score points over bossy solid nurses in clumping shoes by arriving in an elegant flowing dress and doing petit-point embroidery. On no account wear a personal stereo or you will miss the magic moment when they mumble your name, and have to wait another hour.
- When you do see the consultant, mention how long you waited, if you did. He might like to know, and he has a lot of power in the class-ridden hospital society. Tell him no wonder your blood pressure is up.
- Write down your questions before you go in. Somehow, lying half-naked on a high table being prodded by a strange man in a hurry and a brisk, bored midwife, one tends to forget things. But stay friendly; let the midwife see that you respect his or her experience and opinions as much as the doctor's, if not more.
- If the midwife leaves you alone to take your clothes off, and leaves your notes on the table, for heaven's sake read them. Of *course* it is not snooping.
- If you are really worried, don't hide it. With my second child I was irrationally convinced, near the end that something was wrong; but went through almost the whole of my 32-week appointment with a stiff upper lip. One casual kind word from my consultant, just as he was leaving after the regulation 45-second prod, brought on a flood of tears. It saved the day. Back he

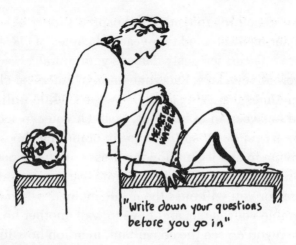

"Write down your questions
before you go in"

came, ordered the nurses to fetch a loudspeaker so that
I could hear Rose's heartbeat, gave me a kick-chart to
fill in, and sent me home to the first peaceful night's
sleep for weeks. The dreadfully businesslike and
abrupt manner of medical people sometimes creates a
sense that they are hiding some awful secret from you.
In fact, they are just brooding about their next pay rise
and whether gorgeous Dr Gupta in Intensive Care really
meant it about the Nurses' Home dance on Friday.

- Read all the books about pregnancy and birth that you
can bear to. Go to classes run by the National
Childbirth Trust if you can. If you can use terms like
placenta, membranes, engagement, cervix and so on,
the staff might talk to you almost as an equal. It is
roughly the same principle you use for outfacing a
contemptuous young garage mechanic who keeps going
on about tappet-adjustments.

- If they won't talk to you, fight. It is often the youngest
doctors who behave most like pigs. Remember all the

time whose baby it is. Here is a piece of dialogue from my own past:

JUNIOR DOCTOR *(bustling in)*: Mrs, erm, er, Heiney. Er. *(addressing midwife).* Is this one complaining of any problems?
ME: A bit of a problem with heartburn and bad leg cramps.
MIDWIFE: She has heartburn and leg cramps, doctor.
JD *(still to midwife)*: Oh. Yes *(scribbles prescription).* Give her that *(tries to depart).*
ME: Hang on, doctor, sorry, what is this prescription for?
JD *(as if suddenly noticing me)*: You just take it to a chemist and he will give you some medicine *(tries to depart again).*
ME: I will bloody well not take it to a chemist. I will take it to my GP and ask *him* for a civil answer. Why should I take anything when you won't even spare me thirty seconds to say whether it's supposed to be for the heartburn or the legs?
(Doctor departs, but his ears are becoming satisfyingly red.)
MIDWIFE: Oh, I am sorry about him. But what can we do?

Such little playlets are being played out every day around the antenatal clinics of the nation. Just make sure your part is a speaking one. And don't worry about making enemies; at least the fragmentation of care in Britain means that you may never see the same doctor or nurse twice, let alone be delivered by anyone whose name you even know. So you can stand up for yourself without much risk of meeting your adversary the next time in advanced labour. If you do, you could always brazen it out and say, 'Oh, how lovely that it's you, someone I know.'

Of course, it would be better not to have any fights at all. I am just saying that if you do, it probably isn't your fault, and I hope you win.

- Finally – a useful hint for staying happy during hospital appointments. Don't watch *ER*, *Casualty* or *Holby City*. In recent years it would seem that the production team of the latter programme has invested in a rather expensive bit of kit which simulates a womb, for filming Caesarean operations. As a result, every other plotline involves an emergency Caesarean, often involving death, mayhem, or the discovery that the baby is an IVF error or product of adultery, because it is entirely the wrong colour. Do yourself a favour, watch *Friends* instead.

As to the *usual physical discomforts of pregnancy*, there are a few things to be done, but most of them too often repeated to be worth enumerating again. At one stage in my childbearing career I decided that if one more kind person told me to eat a slice of bread before getting up (for the sickness), stand properly (for the backache) and take Milk of Magnesia for the heartburn, I would knock them down and sit on them. One acquaintance of mine swears blind that raspberry-leaf tea cures sickness, backache, heartburn and cramps in the legs, and that gipsy women who drink it never have difficult labours. The fact that it tastes like shredded lorry-tyres is neither here nor there.

There are a few things, however, that I wish I had known earlier:

Sickness
If you are, you are. The usual remedies may not work. If you are going to go on throwing up, at least you can manage it gracefully; embarrassment and tension are worse than the actual puking. Get everyone to save you clean airline and coach sick-bags, and carry a stock, with rubber bands to seal them, a damp flannel, and a few tissues. Try to retain a sense of humour when people in the street think that you are a drunk. If you throw up your breakfast, there is no harm in eating another one, to stop you feeling rotten later on. I once had three breakfasts, two unsuccessfully, and presented a live radio programme at nine o'clock. Curiously, going live on the radio completely cured the sickness, as it does hiccups.

Heartburn at night
Cured by sleeping with your shoulders propped up on four pillows, like El Cid lashed upright stone-dead on his horse. But:

Leg cramps
Leg cramps are best cured by having your legs propped up on another four pillows. You feel like a banana. The other cure for leg cramps is to have a sleeping partner trained to fling himself on your calves at the slightest moan and begin massaging the lump away. Mine was so

well-conditioned after two pregnancies that he hurled
himself at my legs if I so much as turned over in the night.

Above all, forget occasionally that you're pregnant. In my
first pregnancy, I had all the above symptoms and more,
but went off sailing, walking round Ushant, and on a fortnight's trip down the Mississippi for a newspaper, travelling hard, hitching rides on towboats and tugs, and
walking alone round the Vieux Carré of New Orleans at
seven months gone. Interestingly, every single symptom
vanished for the duration of the trips. As soon as I got
home, every single one came back.

There are some useful things you can do during a first
pregnancy, although really the best activities are travel,
taking holidays and earning extra money, all of which will
get difficult after the birth. If you must do useful things,
you *could* make detailed preparations, trimming cradles
and laying out tiny vests, even buying nappies. I couldn't
bear to do this; it seemed too much like counting your
chickens before they hatch. I preferred to lie in hospital
while my poor husband went flying around to stock up on
zinc-and-castor-oil cream and bolt the wobbly old cradle
back together. If you share my superstitious dread, but still
feel a need to be doing something and getting in control of
the future, there are a few general things to do, make, and
consider without tempting fate by assuming good luck in
Month Nine. Here they are:

Consider your house
Or flat. Is it warm? Is it easy to get warm? Are there bits of
it where you spend a lot of time, like the kitchen, which

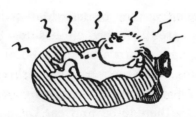

are always cold and draughty? If so, is the cold area close to a warm area where the baby can doze in its basket or sit in a chair watching you?

Is your home a pleasant place to be all day long, or just somewhere you have always flopped after a day's work? You may not want to decorate a nursery, but it pays off handsomely to decorate your main rooms and landings and bathroom. At no other time, probably, will you spend so much time in your own home as when you have a new baby.

Give up any idea that a baby is a small thing which takes up little space. The amount of equipment that accumulates around the most economically run infant is prodigious. It certainly needs a whole chest of drawers to itself. Do you have any storage space to spare? No? Right, what are you going to throw out?

Consider your transport
If you have a car and are about to change it, it might pay to go for a four-door model. The grip that even the tiniest baby can get on the pillar of a two-door car, when you are trying to manoeuvre it into its seat, takes some believing.

Consider your clothes
Maternity clothes should no longer be much of a problem. All the old grumbles about viscose sacks with 'touches of

interest at the neck' are out of date. Mail-order firms and specialists have pretty, folksy clothes for those whose instincts in pregnancy turn a bit more floral than before. High-street chains and XL shops have T-shirts and draw-string pants in a huge range of sizes, which will do for all but the largest mothers-to-be to wear casually at home; saris, kaftans and wild ethnic drapes are fun for evenings and will furnish the future family dressing-up box. It pays to have one really nice pashmina.

A working wardrobe can be more troublesome if your office is formal. Specialist maternity shops provide trouser suits and boring coat-dresses which will help, but if you spend too much money you will resent it. One of the best answers is to borrow off friends or relatives: a particularly fetching Popeye sweatshirt and a lovely striped cotton maternity blazer I know of have draped five babies in three families, including two of mine. The journalist Valerie Grove mistily remembers one tent-dress by Monsoon which got used in eight pregnancies (various incumbents) around literary North London in the 1970s, and finally fell to bits on her sister in Sydney, Australia. Publisher Helen Fraser mysteriously mentions the virtues of 'army surplus', raising an intriguing picture of lumber-ing camouflage printed guerrillas moving in on a mater-nity ward like an overweight platoon of the SAS. A BBC researcher drove half her department wild by simply getting out her old school gymslip (she was a tubby 12-year-old who turned into a slim swan) and flouncing around like an extra in a blue St Trinians film.

You may have trouble with bras: if you start off small-breasted, you are just as well off buying larger and larger sizes of good conventional bras, but if you start off at 38 or so, you will fall prey to the nursing-bra trade. Most nursing bras are profoundly depressing, droopy, misshapen and punitively uncomfortable, and drive you half-mad with frustration and gloom. The ones marketed by the National Childbirth Trust are a bit better – at least you can try them on and exchange by post, and not trudge mournfully around every cubicle in town trying to fit your twin Zeppelins into something bearable.

But on the whole, as I say, maternity clothes are not a problem. Apart from official maternity wear, there are floppy smocks, homemade tents, large-size men's tracksuits and sailing sweaters, husbands' jeans worn with huge safety-pins, and all the 'ethnic' flowing cottons. Those who do best are cheerful, stylish women who can take a joke. The important thing is to accept that you are what you are – pregnant. You don't need to look sexy or

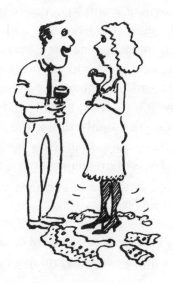

alluring. Clean shiny hair, clear bright colours and a pleasant smile will do, It's not for long.

Once the baby is born, you have definite needs which it pays to anticipate. Make sure you have washable things; forget the dry-clean only culture – it'll break your heart, and your bank. You need smocky tops that push up from the waist for feeding (a good costume for the first few weeks, with or without a winter sweater, is your favourite old cotton maternity shirt worn loose over trousers – then baby can be sick on it without ruining a sweater). Before you go to hospital, it pays to put a few easy, practical clothes together at home in a place where you can find them quickly. I used to long for some simple garment like a Babygro to haul myself into: a Mummygro. With feet.

One final point on clothes: I used to get very cross at tights which crept gradually down over the bump, even if labelled 'maternity'. When I asked my friends what they did (I told you pregnant women get pretty intimate in their conversations), I found that everyone had the same problem. Some switch to socks; one used over-the-knee stockings with garters, and got varicose veins from it; several wore a size larger and put them on back-to-front (swivelling the feet, which is not terribly comfortable) and another simply cut the tights down the front and wore knickers on top. (Like Superman. *Now* we know what was wrong with him! He was pregnant!)

Consider the baby's clothes

If you did nothing at all about these before the birth, you could still send your friend or husband down to the corner chemist to buy five all-in-one suits and five vests, and survive

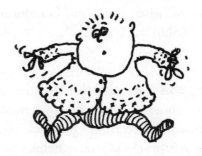

perfectly well for several weeks with a new baby, just adding disposable nappies and a warm little blanket. If you have knitting grannies, aunties and well-wishers, it would help to steer them on to something actually useful: lacy cardigans are terrible, because the baby gets its fingers caught in the holes; most cardigans have far too narrow sleeves for easy dressing, anyway. Wide, loose-armed square sweaters are simpler, and quite smart; best of all is to set the knitters to making a supply of tank-tops (sleeveless slipovers).They look wonderful in stripes, pastel or bright; you can drag them on in seconds over a Babygro, or pyjamas, or another sweater, just to keep the baby a bit warmer without the ordeal of sleeves.

If you find a good source of secondhand clothes to lend or buy, hang on to it!

Finally, **consider your duty**
The responsibility of a baby can seem huge, vague and impossible at times. Too much reading about infant care and bonding and imprinting and early influence can stampede you into a tearful panic. It can depress you into feeling that life will be a dreary round of nappy-changing and fiddling around with sterilizers, broken only by earnest coffee mornings with other sick-stained Mums in a litter

of hideous toys. Clinics hand out leaflets about parent-hood, carrying frightful 'Specimen Daily Routines' like this one:

0630   Mother gives baby early feed, settles baby.
Prepares nourishing breakfast for husband and self. Rinses out overnight nappies, pegs to dry.
0730   Mother eats breakfast, feeds baby, loads washing machine, changes Napisan, cleans kitchen, prepares vegetables for midday meal.

and so on, all day, with never a line suggesting: 'Mother reads paper, walks round garden, goes out and gets hair-cut, goes to drunken lunch with friend.' It is fatally easy to confuse the baby with the bathwater: daily routines, crossover vests, coffee mornings and the peeling of nour-ishing vegetables for husbands are all no more than bath-water. All that is *really* going to happen is that you will become responsible for a small, highly entertaining, amaz-ingly tolerant and self-contained person. Your only duty is to keep this person fed, clean, warm and entertained. There is no reason why you should stay in the house, iron-ing sheets or baking like a 'real' mother, if you don't want to. New babies are completely portable, and care very little where they doze and wake and feed, as long as you are there. Things will change later, but by then you will be expert enough to adjust matters to suit yourself. It is pretty rare for a normal, sober, undrugged woman to do a baby any actual harm; as long as it is fed and clean and warm and has a place to sleep in peace, it will do fine, and prob-ably not even cry much.

Incidentally, if you have doubts about whether you will love your baby, because you think other people's children are horrid, squirmy, snotty, damp pink things, do not worry. It is quite possible to have babies of your own (sweet-smelling, perfect and brilliant) and still perceive other people's as revolting and dull. Nature is very crafty. And the actual tasks of babycare are not bad at all, once a real baby is involved; you may be repelled by 'parentcraft' classes with a grinning plastic doll and frayed terry nappies, yet really enjoy bathing and changing a real, kicking baby of your own.

Your baby's father needs to know all these things, too. He may be feeling as uncertain, excited and nervous as you are. I have deliberately kept fathers in the background in this book; not because that is where they ought to be, or where my own husband is, but only because the moments when a mother most needs support are precisely those lonely times when fathers are off somewhere. The office day, the factory day mean long stretches of paternal absence. The promptings of biology mean that in the first year, even the first three years, and even when both parents have jobs, mothers move fast and urgently towards a child's distress even if father happens to be moving that way too (couples in which the father gets up at night to the baby frequently report that the mother lies awake anyway until he gets back). Some inbuilt tolerance seems to make women more patient with whiners and clingers and vandals and food-flingers. But even so, the more closely a father is involved from the start, the more he will enjoy his babies and the less isolated and solely responsible you will feel.

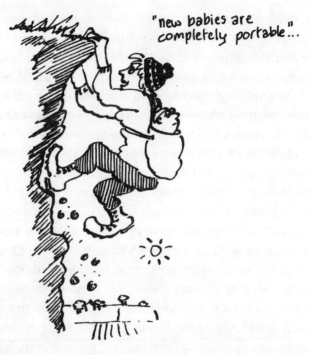

"new babies are completely portable"...

Men do have a different *style* of babycare; I never got a child back from my husband complete with the same number of shoes, socks, hats, gloves, etc. that I handed it over with; but what the hell? Socks are not everything. If he is the sort who baths the baby in hospital, plays, tosses, bounces, gets the first smile to himself, and confidently takes charge of a tiny baby round the clock, then you are lucky and he is lucky and the baby is very lucky indeed. But it doesn't always happen like that; I am writing about under-threes, and some men just can't do much with them, or won't. If that happens, the babies still have to be looked after by someone, and you are the one who is left with no choice. That is why I have written for mothers, about mothers, and with the help of mothers; any father who picks up anything useful from the book is more than welcome, and any father who shoots it down in scorn is, at least, involved. Good luck to him.

If the whole prospect still overwhelms you, do something small and absorbing. Go out, buy some unbreakable fishing line, and restring all your favourite bead necklaces on it. Then you have something the baby can play with and hang on to while you carry it around; and you keep your favourite beads.

Or else earn some extra money, or sell something, and set up a baby fund; there is no time in your life when a few extra pounds will make more difference. One friend combined the problems of no storage and no savings, booked a market stall for a day, looted the house, and made £300 in one afternoon. She still thinks that the sight of a hugely pregnant woman standing on an orange-box shouting her wares ('a sixties Beatle scrapbook ... a personal stereo ... a wok ...') was enough to intimidate the population of South London into buying it all. Besides, it was an adventure. Just because you are about to have The Biggest Adventure of a Woman's Life doesn't mean you can't have a few small ones as well.

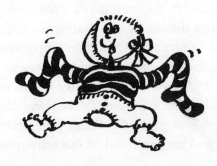

Chapter Two

Hard Labour: Birth

My first child was born in November, when the sellers of Remembrance poppies were out on the streets. I was days overdue; one gloomy evening, my mother-in-law rang for a bulletin. 'Have they come yet,' she enquired lugubriously, 'to take her away?' On being told that they hadn't, her response was electrifying. 'Aye,' she said, generations of old wives' lore quivering in her voice. 'I bought a poppy t'other day. *I thought of Libby.*' And having thus memorably equated my coming confinement with the mud, blood and mortality of the trenches, she left us to wait on, amid the howling winter winds and the chilly fog curling off the river.

We were glad of it, really. It made a nice counterpoint to the breathless optimism of the National Childbirth Trust classes, where an upbeat teacher had stripped away all the mystery from the abdominal events to come, trained us never to refer to 'pain', and generally raised our expectations. We had been comfortably looking forward to a supremely interesting, mildly tiring Life Experience, and it was salutary to be reminded of the other point of view:

the howling, heaving and bedpost-gripping made familiar by a hundred historical novels, and warned of (with graphic hand gestures) by generations of grannies.

For years they told us that when A Woman's Time Has Come, she moans and grips her husband's hand; then comes an interlude of black terror, screaming, sweat, agony and struggle; followed by exhaustion necessitating a month in bed and a ritual visit to the nearest temple for purification of her foulness. Old bags in launderettes still mutter joyfully about Auntie Helen who was Never the Same Again after what she went through with her second; about Our Brenda who never had a day without pain (and it was Twin Beds from the day she came out that hospital until the day *he* passed on, the dirty beast); about dropped bits and ruptured bits and Specialists down from Lunnon who had never seen anything like it in 40 years. The advantage of this great female legend in its heyday was presumably that when the terrified young girls actually came to have babies, they found it nowhere near so bad as they expected; and in their subsequent relief felt positively light-hearted about the few residual aches and pains. The disadvantage was (and is) that the more frightened the mother, the worse it hurts. The legend was thus enabled to live on, with ever more refinements of detail ('Ooh, you should have seen my stitches. I tore *3inches*. Doctor said he'd never seen anything like it ...').

The great legend took a bashing with the advent of the childbirth movement. New childbirth, natural childbirth, Birth without Fear, whatever you call it, the symptoms are much the same. They include a refreshing blast of technical knowledge, a refusal to admit that it hurts much and, at the more extreme limits, the claim by Sheila Kitzinger that 'birth is the most exciting sexual experience of a woman's life' (depends on all the others, I should say ...). The new prophetesses use 'birthing' as an active verb, admire Leboyer's vision of a child drifting into the world to gentle music and dim lights and warm water and love. They point with enthusiasm at Michel Odent's squatting, naked mothers and athletically involved fathers at the Pithiviers clinic, and publish books of exercises to stretch every useful muscle. They write blow-by-blow accounts of their own beautiful labours, surrounded by friends play-ing guitars, nourished by ancient honey-and-raspberry-leaf infusions, and culminating in the joyful eating of the placenta in an iron-rich stew.

This approach, like the other one, has its disadvantages for the nervous, bone-idle, easily confused primagravida. The pursuit of knowledge is useful; being urged to fren-zied activity during labour is a very good thing. (Hospitals ought to have ping-pong tables. At least husbands might, for once, let their wives win as they approach 5 cm dila-tion, and it would be less boring than flinging yourself on a beanbag.) And the scorn poured on painkillers has at least stopped medical staff from their famed practice of shooting women full of pethidine to make them shut up groaning.

On the other hand, all that fulsome praise of Nature tends to infuriate the large minority whose babies, in Nature, would not have had a lot of fun getting out; Caesarean, drip induction, epidural anaesthetic and forceps victims have developed a tendency to complain bitterly about being 'cheated of the experience of birth',

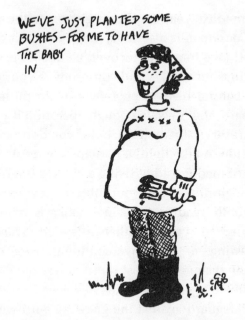

WE'VE JUST PLANTED SOME
BUSHES - FOR ME TO HAVE
THE BABY
IN

which must sound incredible to the howling-and-bedposts school of obstetrical fantasists. Like complaining about being cheated of the rack or the thumbscrew. Almost as bad is the awful guilt, felt by the likes of me, that no baby can have a calm and silently magical Leboyer delivery if the first sound to assail its little slimy ears is the sound of its mother swearing like a Billingsgate porter and punching its father in the neck.

Now, on top of this struggle between the earth-mothers and the doomsters, comes a sneaky but influential lobby which says 'Look, spare yourself the hassle, keep the diary tidy, go for an elective Caesarean.' Earth-mothers, and some doctors, are outraged by the 'too posh to push' lobby; however, you may come under subtle pressure from mothers who chose Caesareans for psychological or social

rather than medical reasons. Don't give in without thinking hard: a Caesarean is a serious, major abdominal operation; you will take longer to recover, be unable to drive or
lift heavy things for weeks, and compromise your chances
of having a natural birth later. Infections, even fatalities,
are not unheard-of. It's a safe enough operation if you need
an op, and preserves many lives; but if you don't need it, it
is not an option to take lightly. Perhaps the most disgraceful example of medical advertising ever was the US ad for
Caesareans beginning 'Keep your tubes honeymoon fresh!'

On the whole, reading 'birthing' books is more useful
than listening to your mother-in-law delivering the
Gypsy's Warning, or your overconfident friends telling
you how their system was best (all mothers have to think
their own choice regarding babies has been best, at every
stage. It's a safeguard against the gnawing guilt we all feel
most of the time. You learn to discount it). When it comes
to choosing which hospital, you can get some good infor-
mation from friends, though, and the underground
network of mothers' groups, and the hearsay evidence of
your classmates at the heavy-breathing sessions. I heard,
this way, that a certain hospital has one obstetrician who
is gay and can't stand the sight of women's breasts; that
another plays country 'n' western muzak in the delivery
rooms (babies' heads, emerging, feel exactly as if they had
concrete Stetsons on anyway, without any such uncomfortable musical suggestion); and that yet another hospital
has a tendency to bring in six medical students at a time to
gaze at your perineum and gasp at your language. (The
woman who told me this had actually raised herself on
her elbows, between pushes, and demanded ticket money

from the growing crowd at her feet. Two of them were so startled they actually began fishing in their white coat pockets.) At least if you know all this, you are prepared.

One awful warning came my way about home births. These are so difficult to organize, for a first baby in Britain, that one couple dedicated two months of lobbying, changing doctors, persuading and campaigning to win permission to be tended at home. Finally they got it; and as soon as the thrill of the chase had worn off, misgivings set in. The woman confided, a little shamefacedly, that in her excitement at beating the system, she never once thought about the work and disruption it would cause – not to the medical staff, but to her own house. On the day she got the official list of things to prepare (like high blocks to put the bed on, and vast quantities of plastic sheeting for the bedroom carpet) she longed to recant, but didn't have the face to. Her husband eventually spent half the delivery night clearing up, and the next morning washing the dozen teacups and biscuit plates emptied by the community midwife (the doctor had most of the Scotch afterwards). Both parents, occasionally, still have wistful thoughts about nice clean hospitals with unlimited laundry and professional tea-ladies.

My own husband, having cheered me on through two hospital deliveries and revelled in the fact that someone else would clear up, now says after ten years of farming that these matters are best carried out in outdoor lambing-pens, with all present in Wellington boots. So, round here, only sheep are allowed home births.

(I should admit, though, that I am not the most impartial person to discuss home births. With my first child, I discovered to my shame that I am a complete hospital junkie; I loved every moment, became institutionalized within two days, had to be dragged out, complaining, at the end of eight days; and for months afterwards, I indulged in yearning fantasies about going back to the lovely maternity ward. One weary night, when Rose was two months old, I announced this longing; my husband asked, 'What is so special about hospital, for heaven's sake?' and I apparently sobbed: 'They bring a trolley of laxatives and sleeping pills round at nine o'clock sharp every night. I never actually *have* anything, but at least it shows that someone cares.' Mystified, the poor man took to offering me a laxative every night, just before the nine

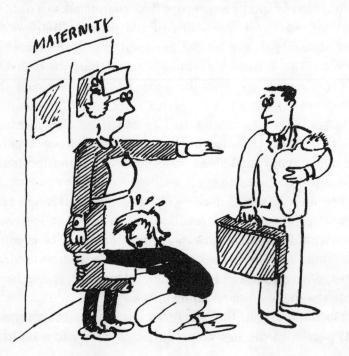

o'clock news, to show he cared; but it wasn't the same, somehow.) But then, I was lucky in my hospitals. Not everybody is; and more recent practice is to chuck the new mother and baby out pretty sharply after the birth, to go through the rest of the recovery stage at home.

So, to the birth itself: every birth is slightly different. All I can usefully say is: beware of Legends, and beware of Irrelevant Campaigns.

Legends

'A woman always knows when she is in labour.'
Oh no, she doesn't. Hospitals get women arriving two minutes from birth, still wondering vaguely if anything is amiss; and countless others turning up a fortnight early with indigestion and nerves. Keep an open mind about it, and don't be too easily fooled by the spectacular Braxton-Hicks contractions which sweep over you while you're watching *Big Brother*.

'Your waters will break, embarrassingly, in the supermarket, with no warning at all.'
Well, they may. Possibly. It is still not worth going around for weeks on a knife's edge of uncertainty, avoiding supermarkets. I drove down for some Sunday papers just before Rose was born, and suddenly found myself sitting on a sodden car-seat. Panicking, I drove carefully home again, feeling false labour pains rack me every two minutes, and shrieked for my husband, for an emergency babysitter for my elder child, for pethidine or a Caesarean or a community midwife or anybody at all. Paul leaped into the

driving-seat, paused, and began to laugh immoderately. '*My* waters have gone as *well*,' he gasped. Before any domestic violence could set in, he explained: someone had left the car window open in the rain overnight; the water had soaked deep into the foam upholstery; the seat was now dry to the touch, but immediately became soaked when someone sat heavily down on it. Strained laughter all round.

'*When you are ready or overdue, you can induce the baby naturally by massaging your nipples.*'

It produces some useful hormone, they say. But only if you do it for several hours. There are few things a hugely pregnant woman feels less like doing than massaging her nipples all day. Take my word for it.

'*A bumpy car ride will bring a baby on.*'

It would have to be very bumpy indeed, if 20 miles round the Lincolnshire back-lanes in a reconditioned Russian army motorcycle sidecar failed to have any effect on my sister-in-law in the 41st week ...

'*When the moment comes, you will feel an overwhelming urge to push.*'

I would never have dared to dismiss this great universal belief until I had my second baby without feeling the remotest wish to push anything at all. Since then, I have met other women and got them to admit it, too. We all pushed our babies out quite efficiently, waiting for contractions and just doing it; but felt no urge, just a sullen boredom with the whole process, and a desire to get it over with. Nobody should be bullied or stereotyped by everybody else's biology.

> *'You will be overwhelmed by love and wonderment at the sight of the baby, newborn and laid on your stomach.'*

Well, you *may* be; once out of two births, I was; the other time I was being sick and fancied a cup of tea more than a slimy baby. This is no tragedy; my husband held both of our newborns straight away, while I got myself together, and there were no ill-effects on any of us. Which leads to the most dangerous legend of all ...

> *'For a mother to hold and suckle her child immediately is essential to the "bonding" of mother and child. If a mother is stopped from doing this, she may suffer postnatal depression and her relationship with the child will not develop.'*

This is an awful thing to say to a mother who may end up under general anaesthetic, or ill herself, or with a desperately sick baby in an incubator. What is she supposed to do? Bond with the tea-trolley instead? Human beings have brains and hearts as well as bodies; it is time the 'bonding' lobby admitted this.

It is an even worse thing to say to a mother who has no medical crisis, but simply doesn't want to hold her baby instantly, after her hours of exhausting labour and months of exhausting pregnancy. Why the hell should she? When my happy, healthy, untroubled baby daughter, now the apple of my eye, was first born I took one look and said, 'My God, it looks like a bloody shark' (which she did:

underslung jaw and peculiar squashed nose). I let my husband do the cooing. After 20 minutes I fed her, quite successfully; then she went to sleep and I was wheeled off to a side ward. The nurses came in agitatedly, to say that my ward was too cold for a newborn, and they couldn't find a heater; could they possibly leave the baby in the warm nursery until morning? Would it upset me? I said no; and Rose's first night, fast asleep, was not spent beside my bed. With the first baby, he and I had lain staring at one another for six hours, wide awake, and that was very nice too, in its way; but as for 'bonding', it made no difference whatsoever. Of course it is unfortunate to take a new baby right off to an incubator or a nursery for hours; but it is just as unfortunate to expect a tired, cross, sleepy woman to put on a big act of instant love for her baby when she doesn't feel like it. Love comes more slowly than that, to many women; you can depress a mother horribly by making her feel like an unmaternal monster for not cooing and staring into the cot all the time.

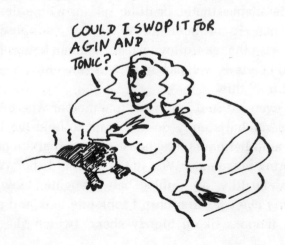

COULD I SWOP IT FOR
A GIN AND
TONIC?

Irrelevant campaigns

No offence intended to the campaigners; but there are certain, once excellent, causes which have become rather bigger than the problems they set about solving. In my first childbirth, I was educated by the pioneering books on natural birth, and fired by the feminist spirit. On my first visit to the clinic, almost my first words to the surprised midwife were, 'I'm not having an enema, you know!' I vowed to chain myself to the hospital railings before I submitted to a shave ('ritual humiliation of women'), I argued about episiotomies when I was only two months gone, and recited statistics on induction and its fearful side-effects to any baffled trainee midwife who would listen. I cornered obstetricians at parties, jeering about foetal heart monitoring and scalp-clips while they tried to spear sausages on toothpicks; I was a terrible, terrible bore.

Quite rightly, I got my come-uppance on the day. For impeccable medical reasons I was induced, put on a drip, and prescribed an epidural anaesthetic to keep my blood pressure down; and a slightly distressed baby was rescued, hale and hearty, by way of a lift-out forceps delivery and an episiotomy. I had the enema and shave quite willingly because I happened to like the rather bawdy, extrovert old midwife who offered them; as for ritual humiliation of women, Sister Hubbard would not have put up with any of that for a minute. (Her own technique of ritual humiliation of arrogant young male doctors on the ward was wonderful to behold.)

The irony is that, when it came to the second birth in a very liberal, natural-childbirth-minded hospital, I spent half my labour saying things like: 'What about an epidural, eh, nurse? Are you sure I shouldn't be shaved? If a little episiotomy would speed things up, I'm sure ... Suppose you broke the waters now, eh, doctor? I'm sure I should have had a colonic irrigation by now ...' In short, I was an even worse bore. I had no anaesthetic at all, except for a happy interlude with the gas-and-air cylinder (a pretty exciting experience for a girl who has gone nine months without a drink); I had a tear instead of an episiotomy, and felt no particular difference afterwards.

The moral of all this is: relax. Or, if you want, *be* a bore. The great thing about childbirth is that it is the last time you can behave appallingly, swear, lay down the law, shriek, groan and bash your husband in the chest, and be forgiven. You are the star, the primadonna; make the most of it. Once the new star arrives, to the sound of your last furious swear-word, you will have to behave again, and be gentle and self-sacrificing. Enjoy your last fling.

Practicalities

Hospitals give you lists of things to bring with you; the one thing never mentioned is paper knickers; or, if you can't find them in the shops, the worst old Mummy-pants in your drawer, to throw away. Take 20 pairs, and you'll never regret it. And however lissome you are, this is absolutely not the moment for thongs. Enough said.

Understandably, hospitals don't encourage you to bring anything much into the delivery room, but various groups like the National Childbirth Trust will recommend amusements and comforts, ranging from sponges to light reading. Here are some less conventional items that women have taken into the delivery room and been glad of:

- A pair of thick woolly socks (hot face, cold feet).
- An aerosol spray of 'Fresh Air'. (One friend says, 'I farted like a mad thing all the way through, very embarrassing smell.' Sorry.)
- A small plastic plant-spray for when your husband gets bored with sponging your face all the time.
- A cassette machine of music. (But beware. Just as the obstetrician approached with his forceps to extract my first, Paul switched on our machine to take my mind off it all, and it happened to be set at a sea song: 'Haul away Joe'. Not very tasteful, but it made the doctor laugh.)
- A camera. (Pictures of your baby at ten minutes old are wonderful. For some reason they look more grown-up than a week later: wise and amused.)
- Lip salve.
- A guitar. (One girl tried to get permission for a Hammond Organ, but failed.)
- A mirror (to watch the head born, if you fancy. I don't).
- *Harpers & Queen.* (Not a magazine I normally read, but Jennifer's Diary, performed in a high posh voice by Paul, kept me laughing immoderately into the gas-and-air mask right up to the start of second-stage labour.) *Hello* or *OK!* magazine would do as well. Nothing serious is going to get through your defences, so don't assume this is the moment to tackle Stephen Hawking for the first time.
- A laptop and a stack of DVD films (if you're that techno-friendly. Anything with Goldie Hawn in it is a good bet, I am told).

- A picnic for afterwards (miss hospital mealtimes and you've had it for six hours).
- A Marybean (tropical seed from the West Indies, believed to be lucky in childbirth).
- A horseshoe (same reason).
- A game of Scrabble. (But one mother reports that it easily gets a bit close to the bone. 'Blood … conception … tubes … then we gave up!')

Above all, or instead of it all:

- A father. If he won't come, he won't, and a girlfriend or sister or mother would do. Better a willing partner than a groggy, reluctant one. But if the baby's father will come, he might surprise you: men are often so good in the labour room, contrary to daft old legends, that the midwives are lost in admiration. (It can go too far, even. The young nurse breathed admiringly to me, after Rose was born, 'Your husband is wonderful. Anyone would think he had been at dozens of confinements.' I replied, a little sourly, that this was unlikely. Unless he has a hobby of which I know nothing. Perhaps he slips on a white coat and creeps into maternity wards on his days off.)

Afterword

The days in hospital with a newborn, and the first fragile week back home, are a strange, limbo-like time. Selfishness is absolutely essential. Don't keep trying to please everyone; it's your time. If you don't want a diffi-cult relative to visit you, say so. One girl, who had lost a baby at four days, had suffered all through her second pregnancy from her mother-in-law's insinuations about genetic defects ('If it happens once, it'll happen again'). She was frantic to keep this dreadful old bag away, at least for five or six days; but had been advised by all sorts of well-meaning professionals that hospital visiting was vital to 'family bonding'. I am afraid I sneakily advised her to hold her ground, and, if necessary, ban her own mother as well, just to even things out diplomatically.

Accepting help is also essential. Independent, strong, healthy women feel stupid at being brought meals in bed and having their babies' nappies changed by nurses, or back home by kindly sisters-in-law or paid maternity nurses. But take advantage. If you looked around in an old-fashioned hospital where mothers stay in for several days, you could always tell the first- from second-time mothers on a ward; all the novices would be struggling tearfully with the fifth nappy of the morning, sticking pins in themselves and annoying the baby, just to prove they can cope. Meanwhile the old lags lie back on their pillows, murmuring, 'Well, sister, I do have a little backache, if you'd be terribly kind and change him I'd be so grateful ...' They don't have to prove that they can cope alone. They've done it. Anyway, *everybody,* except the very subnormal, can cope alone eventually, tough though it may be. Why start work early when you could be lying back eating grapes and cuddling a nice, clean, changed baby? If you feel ropey, are incontinent, in pain from stitches, piles, sore nipples, engorgement or whatever, it will pass; there is no point in feeling that you have to win your maternal spurs now, in the first couple of days, by changing every nappy.

By the way, bursting into tears on Day Five is so common a phenomenon that nobody who looks after new mothers is remotely surprised by it. But don't time your most unnerving and demanding visitors for Day Five, and tell your partner in advance that it may happen, and does not mean that you are sinking into the lowest abysses of real post-natal depression.

The only thing worth fighting about, in hospital, is demand-feeding. These days you rarely even have to fight for it. Appalling though it may seem to feed a baby every 45 minutes round the clock (each feed lasting 15 minutes ... or more ...), if that is what it wants, then that is the best thing to give it. It keeps the baby from crying, and speeds up the moment when it will feed at sensible times (the more sucking, the more milk). Top-ups of formula are no help at all. But because you are demand-feeding, which is the most supremely unselfish action one human being routinely does for another, you are entitled to be as selfish as hell for the rest of the time. Consider yourself, for a few days. Insist on comfort, rest and peace. Take advantage. Lean on everybody. The baby, after all, is leaning on you. Hard.

• •

Basket Babies:
Infancy

Everything was ready in the tiny flat. The slight matrimonial tension which had blown up over the wine-rack had now abated (the baby was to sleep in the dining-room, and while the books prescribe a temperature of 68°F for babies, wine needs to be cooler. *She* had favoured letting the wine take its chance; *he* favoured putting the baby to bed in a woolly hat and snowsuit. Eventually they moved the wine). Suddenly, up to their door came the Health Visitor, prim and smiling, her alert little eyes roving everywhere. My pregnant friend welcomed her, all unsuspiciously, made her a cup of tea, and sat down anxiously to listen to whatever advice might be forthcoming.

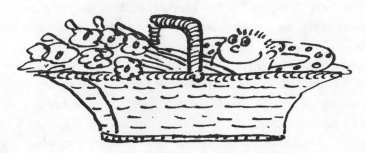

'Now, Mrs D_____ ' said the lady in uniform, with that offensively breezy confidence so often displayed by child-less twenty-two-year-old health professionals towards anxious primagravidae ten years their senior; 'are you planning to use terry nappies, or disposables?'

'Good God, disposables, of course,' said the mother-to-be, startled. Moving the wine-rack was one thing – compromises have to be made, after all – but dabbling around all day in a bucketful of wet sewage was quite another matter. Out of the question.

The health visitor smiled indulgently, making a note.

'Disposables,' she said. 'Well, Mrs D_____ ' (another terrible smile), *'you mustn't feel at all guilty about that, you know.'*

My unfortunate friend, into whose cheerfully optimistic picture of motherhood the idea of guilt had never yet intruded, was struck dumb. Guilt suddenly loomed on the horizon, glowing like a nightmare moon, illuminating every aspect of parenthood with rays of uncertainty and fear. Over the coming weeks hospitals and grannies, doctors and strangers and sisters-in-law and so-called friends would combine to intensify that gloomy and deceptive light. (Actually, there are now so many high-tech terry nappies on the market, and in urban areas so many nifty nappy services, that this particular issue is no longer such a hot one. But the point is the health visitor's use of the G-word.)

You can be made to feel guilty about not using terry nappies; if you do use them, guilty about their being a bit grey after a couple of washes. You can be made to feel guilty about bottle-feeding, and even about breastfeeding

('Poor little chap, he's hungry again, are you sure you've got enough?'). Guilt lies in wait behind the bathroom door ('Of course, I always use cotton wool on their poor little bottoms, with warm boiled water, not those horrid chilly chemical baby wipes'). It haunts the chest of drawers ('These modern clothes are terribly easy for the mother, of course, but their poor little bottoms could at least *breathe,* in the days when they wore pure wool leggings'). Guilt can hover when the baby cries, yet pounce when you pick it up for comfort ('Making a rod for your own back, dear, spoiling that child – it isn't the kindest thing, in the long run'). Guilt squats down in the kitchen, watching you tearfully wrenching the lids off baby-food jars ('Not very like real food, is it?'). Guilt peers at your baby lying quietly in his basket ('Poor old chap, a bit boring for you, isn't it? They do say that understimulation slows them down later'), but it clicks its tongue disapprovingly when you prop him up to watch you round the kitchen ('Well, it's a lot of strain on their poor little backs, of course, with the bones so soft'). To resist the sense of guilt entirely, you have to become a sort of John Wayne of motherhood: tough, opinionated, self-confident and contemptuous of the world. Outlaw Mum, ridin' her own trail. Alternatively, you just have to take a long calm look at your baby, and realize that despite your many shortcomings, *it is perfectly all right.* It likes you. It is cleanish, and not particularly hungry just now. It takes life as it comes. The fact that it is also wearing a paper nappy, odd socks and one of its two-year-old brother's sweaters rolled up to the elbows is irrelevant. So is the fact that it is sitting propped on sofa-cushions in a cardboard box, watching

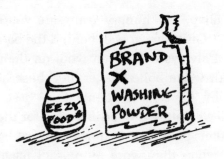

MTV, and hasn't been weighed at the clinic for weeks. (I took my first baby down there religiously once a week, and filled in a chart recording every ounce and centimetre of growth. But the second one did not see a set of scales after she was four weeks old and is thriving to this day. Both ways, though, I was really pleasing myself: I *liked* clocking up the pounds on the first baby, and ignored rude suggestions that I was 'a bit over-fussy, it does no good in the end, you know'. With the second baby I just didn't feel like it, and any fool could see she was healthy, so I didn't do it. When a brief pang of guilt returned and made me murmur to the health visitor that perhaps I ought to bring Rose down to the clinic soon, she – a genuine, card-carrying parent – just said, 'Oh, don't be silly. Look at her!')

The important thing about new babies is that they don't want much; but what they do want, they want *very fiercely*. And there is no point whatsoever in making them wait for it. They will only get crosser and crosser, make you furious yourself, and eventually get so upset that they don't want whatever it was any more, but only to scream with rage for half an hour. It seems incredible, but there are qualified hospital sisters and experienced mothers (presumably amnesiacs) who still say things like 'The baby's got to learn who's master – leave him to cry,' and who advocate strict four-hourly feeding even for brand new babies who have never heard of clocks. Some even talk smugly about 'a nice strong pair of lungs' while a red-faced furious infant shrieks defiance in their bland, stupid faces. All this discipline and learning-who's-the-boss comes much later; what these morons have forgotten is the time-scale of babyhood. A newborn is not a six-week-old who can be distracted from food with rattles; a six-week-old is not a crawler; nor is a crawler much like a wilful two-year-old. It takes nearly two years before a baby actually gets clever enough to 'try it on' or play power games with you. If you start to ascribe older children's motives and morals to a young baby, you are going to be driven mad. To its mother, a baby's crying is a dreadful sound. (Interestingly, it is less dreadful to everyone else. I have sat in friends' houses and had a mother apologize for the background mewling of her baby when I hadn't even noticed it. To her, it was a deafening torment.) So for your own sake, short of smothering or drugging, anything which stops a baby from crying is a good idea.

I have made breakfast while dancing around the kitchen with a Sooty glove-puppet on one hand, singing 'Paper Roses' in a forced baritone, to stop a wakeful son grizzling with boredom at three weeks old. I have sat in the bath with the Moses basket positioned under the towel-rail and a mobile hung above it, swiping the string with the loofah once a minute to keep the butterflies moving and the baby interested and quiet. I have fed at thirty-five-minute intervals all around the clock and have let a new baby suck at the breast for a whole hour; I have made weird squeaking noises in crowded railway carriages to distract a two month-old daughter. I have actually resorted to changing an infant's clothes unnecessarily twice in an afternoon, just because the said infant seemed to find it entertaining. All mothers, and many fathers, do these mad things just to stop the crying. They have to, because even the smallest babies want more than food and sleep: they want entertainment and company. 'It is the central crucial fact of early motherhood', said a journalist friend bitterly, 'that all is well, until you want to do something else.' That cross little blob, eyes only just open, is as avid for amusement as any Broadway boulevardier or teenage raver. Nor will he be fobbed off for long with the old stand-bys, like dangly mobiles and musical-boxes. I asked a collection of mothers and fathers to be honest about how they had amused small babies too young to hold rattles.

The methods included:

- Watching dancing flames (fires have been lit in July for this purpose alone).
- Lying under washing-lines (clean clothes have been strung up, indoors, just for babies to watch).
- Watching budgies ('Only you must have two, so they are active and noisy enough').
- Looking at Op Art patterns in books. (At last, a use for the 1960s. New babies are programmed to be more interested in complicated things than in the simple, bold patterns which toddlers enjoy. Something to do with enabling them to enter a complex world.)
- Putting the carrycot on a washing-machine on fast spin (mind it doesn't vibrate off).

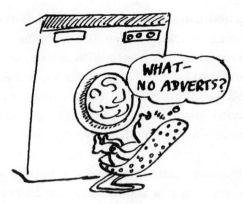

- Propping the baby up in a lean-back seat to watch kitchen activity, front-loading washing-machines, or just about anything. (I have long thought that a lean-back seat with a slowly revolving turntable might find a market.)
- Taking them for a drive round and round the block in the car.
- Tying balloons everywhere (the whole process, from blow to pop, so fascinates babies of all ages that every mother ought to carry a pocketful, or get them in the Bounty Bag at the hospital).
- Shouting football chants along with the baby (a man's solution).
- Giving the cat an extra-strong catnip mouse to go mad with, and propping the baby up to watch.
- Once an interest in toes develops, you can win minutes of peace by simply whipping off their socks and revealing all.

And if all else fails, the best safeguard is the old one, of a huge family and floating population of friends. An alert, short-tempered baby will be at its best at Christmas, and relish adoring uncles, cousins, neighbours, postmen, anybody. If you fill the house with guests, or travel and visit, the work you do will actually be no harder; you just replace loofah-mobile-swiping and trying to cook with the baby balanced on one hip, with walking to bus-stops or making tea for the guests who have mercifully taken over the baby.

Parties are even better, because you eat grown-up food that somebody else has cooked and don't have to do the washing-up. Many an infant's first memories have included a great teetering pile of coats, as it woke in its carrycot in the spare room with a party going on next door. When my son was four weeks old, he had only been to three places in his life: hospital, home and the Olympia Horse Show. We had friends with a box, and permanent guest tickets, and the baby's godfather John Parker was driving his coach-and-four in the final tableau and taking a team of Hungarian greys through an avenue of fire. So every single night I set off across London with the basket, wearing a loose-fitting lurex top to combine the constant feeding with a gesture towards glamour; and every night, in the box, Nicholas lay in state while friendly drunken Scotsmen lurched up to press lucky pound notes into his fist. He smiled at everyone, fed contentedly, and dozed off while Dorian Williams bawled his commentary on the show-jumping across the vast arena below. 'Thank God,' the baby seemed to be saying, his beady eyes swivelling busily around the scene, 'someone has at last understood my requirements.' All he had ever wanted, to keep him passably amused, was ten thousand people, four military bands, two hundred horses and a boxful of tipsy admirers.

At home, in contrast, we had dreadful evenings: trying to read or watch television while the baby struggled against sleep, grizzled, sucked endlessly and finally flaked out at midnight, two hours past our ideal adult bedtime. I think he was missing Olympia.

Another great advantage of handing new babies around to everybody ('The milk bill? Ah, yes, I'll just find the money – take the baby, would you?') is that new babies need to be talked to. And you may not feel like doing it. Next to the section on 'bonding' in the baby books, there is generally a paean of praise for mothers who talk all the time to their babies, maintain 'eye contact', allow infants to study their faces endlessly, and stick out their tongues to test reflexes. This is fine, when you have the time and if you are fortunate enough to have developed an instant adoration of the baby. If you are busy, or tired, or depressed at your life with this unsmiling little creature which gives nothing back and wakes you up four crippling times a night, the task of chatting to it may loom as unwelcome as all the other hundred jobs you have to do in your twenty-four-hour day. Despite underlying love, I hated talking to my second child for nearly two months; she never smiled until then, and I was exhausted, ill and in constant jealous demand from the older child. So I just fed the baby, then encouraged my husband or anyone else in sight to take her over. In the end, they taught her to smile; and then she smiled at me, and taught me in turn to enjoy her company. This, according to the bonding lobby, is disgraceful behaviour. She should have been 'recognizing my voice from her womb experience' and making a 'passionate and exclusive' relationship with me. Ah well. She made a passionate and *in*clusive relationship with everyone in sight, instead; which is probably why at 18 she is the life and soul of every party and plans to go on the stage.

There are a hundred baby-maintenance manuals telling you every detail of how to care for infants physically. I will not bore you with another treatise on nappy-folding and how to dry a baby on your lap. (I have never managed this latter skill, anyway. I think nurses must have very, very long lower-legs, or specially designed chairs. I always end up crouched on the floor over a changing-mat as I anxiously count the bendy little fingers emerging from each woolly sleeve.)

But, backed up by a trusty panel of sick-stained advisers, I can offer a few observations from the heart.

Feeding

Let nobody kid you that breastfeeding is not going to be hell at first. The mammary lobbyists are so keen to promote 'breast is best' (well, it is) that many of them have tended to slide rather dishonestly over the discomfort and exhaustion of the first weeks. Consequently, I suspect, a lot of willing mothers give up, convinced that they are rare cases who 'can't do it'. And indeed, anyone with throbbing, bleeding nipples, dreadful heavy swollen red bosoms, sharp needling letdown pains and a baby who still demands feeding every hour and a half at six weeks old, is entitled to any tantrum she cares to throw. I remember waking my husband up at 3 a.m. one painful morning with the words, 'Shall I tell you something? I *hate* bloody

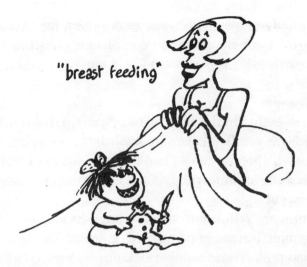

"breast feeding"

breastfeeding, that's what!' There are many paintings of the Madonna and Child, but in none of these has the feeding Madonna got her teeth clenched and her toes curled, as the dreadful infant mouth takes its first agonizing drag.

However, the awful stage usually does end; sometimes in a week or two, sometimes not for a couple of months. And when breastfeeding becomes automatic, it is wonderful. Breast *is* best. Healthiest, safest, least likely to produce an ailing or obese child. It is also very convenient. If you persevere, 'phoning your National Childbirth Trust breastfeeding counsellor in the middle of the night, refusing to listen to anyone who suggests 'just a little formula to top him up', and generally holding out against all adversity like an early Christian martyr being mauled by a small but determined lion, the day will arrive when you can go anywhere with the baby tucked in a basket, and only a couple of spare nappies for equipment. My daughter never even had a drink of water for four months; didn't want it.

Everybody knows that breast milk is best for babies in every way; but here are seven completely selfish reasons why breastfeeding is best for mothers too:

- It's cheaper.
- It's less bother in the end. No boring sterilizing-routine, no powdery milk all over the kitchen, no worrying about whether the rubber teat is fast or slow or blocked; no messing around with hot and cold thermoses when you go out.
- Nappies are yellow and smell quite pleasantly of cinnamon, instead of being hard, green and foul on bottled milk. The inevitable sick-ups also smell better.
- You can go anywhere as long as the baby goes too. Later, you can always express a feed and even have a stock of frozen breast milk. When I was working at the *Tatler* I used to pump off 8 oz with a cylindrical hand-pump (the best sort; avoid all pumps that look like early motor-horns) and I would store it in the editorial fridge all afternoon next to the Art Editor's champagne. Then I took it home, and Nicholas had it for his lunch the next day, while I pumped off the next lot ten miles away in the office Ladies'. This went on from the fourth to the ninth month, and not entirely for his sake, either. It was so that I could go back to full breastfeeding three times a day at weekends, and not have to make up fiddly bottles when we were off sailing.
- You always have an infallible way of shutting the baby up, even during teething. Teeth are no deterrent: one of mine had nearly a full set before I stopped. The only time I got bitten, I took the child off, glared hard at its

rosy little face, and said, 'Never again, sunshine, or it's the bottle for you.' Even at six months, the message seemed to sink in.

- The baby doesn't seem to get so much wind. Wind is a *very* boring business, not least because every old bat who presumes to advise you is an alleged expert on it, and puts down every cross grizzle to either 'teething' or 'wind'. She then springs on the baby and rubs its back ferociously, cupping its chin with a finger and thumb. Later, the baby farts thankfully, alone in its cot. Both my breastfed babies were almost entirely self-winding.

- Thanks to your precious antibodies, immunities etc., the baby is less likely to get frightening and exhausting childhood illnesses while it is very small. They say that most of the immunities are actually passed on in the first couple of weeks, in the colostrum. But there must be something in the later milk which wards off ailments; literally dozens of feeders I have met say that their babies 'got their first cold' a fortnight after the last feed.

I might add to the list the theory that breastfeeders lose weight faster. However, it is not necessarily true. I only began to lose any when I stopped, and a rather reluctant GP admitted that this is not rare. Still, who cares? After all, you're probably not much of a sex object anyway, with those bags under your eyes.

Above all, a splendid reason to breastfeed is that it dispels 90 per cent of that dreary guilt. It absolutely silences criticism. Whatever anybody may think of your chaotic house, grey nappies, commercial baby-jars and nasty modern push-chairs ('A pram rests their poor little backs, and keeps those horrid draughts out, but then these days it's the mothers' convenience that seems to count, dear, isn't it?'), they have to admit that you are giving the brat the best start possible. And you have to admit it to yourself, too. It is a great ego-booster, in principle: and in practice, the prolactin hormone which it sends coursing through your veins after a few months' feeding can be as good as a double gin any day.

As for feeding in public, I admit to being entirely shameless about it. I loathe seeing a baby on a train or a bus, wailing miserably and rooting around in its mother's clothes, while she blushes and soothes and gets crosser and hotter by the minute. The pair of them ought to get on with it, and feed. One of mine has had the right breast in the Terminal 1 departure lounge at Heathrow, and the left breast during takeoff; both of them enjoyed peaceful sessions on many an Inter-City train at 125 miles an hour, and I never, never allowed myself to be discreetly shuffled off to 'a quiet bedroom upstairs' at a party, shut away from company and drink. I have fed bravely in front of gay bachelors, bishops and every shade of prude; I have laughed along with ribald old Yorkshiremen on station platforms saying, 'Eh, poor little lad! He'll never eat all *that!*' and falling about at their own wit. I have only once met a miserable sod who tutted and clucked at my discreet feeding, and by then I had gained enough chutzpah to put it to him straight: 'All right, squire, which is it to be? Screaming, or feeding? You choose.'

Because, of course, you *can* be discreet. The knack is to wear a loose sweater and push it up from the waist, so that the baby itself covers any frightening flesh. Front-opening dresses and bras are a bit of a disaster, in public; shawls are all very well, but require the skill of a handkerchief dancer, especially if an ecstatic little fist gets a grip on them. The main thing to remember is that if *you* are happy, so will everyone else be, and if they're not, they're sick. My brother, the father of two, begged me to quote a typical man's point of view (no hippie, either, but a provincial solicitor shrouded from head to toe in hairy tweeds). 'Don't hide it, don't flaunt it,' he says, 'just do it. You're unlikely to offend anyone you'd *like*.'

Having said all that, I must confess that I have never fed at the table, at least not anyone else's table; and that there is some truth in my colleague Helen's vulgar observation that 'While *you* see the baby's dear little face nuzzling up, what *they* see is acres of boob and a huge nipple bouncing around.' Actually, once my babies reached about six months, and started to beam and wave at everybody, I became more secretive about feeding. There is something slightly indelicate about a baby taking a huge swig from the breast, twisting its head around, and giving the rest of the carriage a big knowing grin. The other passengers feel unable to laugh at the baby without appearing to laugh at ... er, the rest. This struggle can contort their faces painfully, and make you go red. But for the first four or five months, the baby concentrates hard, and all is well. And after that, there are other things you can use to ward off howling; rattles and rusks and the like.

All that I would add, from one bitter experience, is that if you start to feed a baby on a train, unbuttoning, shawl-pulling, unhooking, arranging and settling like a fluffy hen amid folds of fabric and snuffling little gurgles and enthu-siastically waving woolly legs – just make sure that you know where your ticket is, that's all. Men in peaked hats, tapping their toes impatiently, can seriously disarrange your clothing.

Whether you breast- or bottle-feed, however, there is one other thing that I would say: do not dream of expect-ing a 'pattern' to emerge for at least three months. If it does, congratulations. You have a pleasingly clockwork baby. But if any of us were to chronicle the false patterns, the lulls, the storms of perpetual feeding, the general loony and uncontrollable eating behaviour of a new baby, it would be impossible to make a sensible theory out of it. The only thing which seems to help is to institute 'lunch', so that the day falls into two halves. There may be three feeds before 'lunch', and one after, and vice versa the next day; but at least if you call it lunch, you are expressing your faith that one day a sensible and workable routine will evolve. Which it will. The only thing which helped me through the chaos of the early months of demand-feed-ing was determinedly not thinking of the baby as a person (in respect of feeding) because it would be such a capri-cious, unreasonable person that it would drive me crazy. Instead, I thought of him as a sort of *weather*: a little, unpredictable microclimate. You don't expect it to rain at 9.30 today just because it did yesterday, do you? Well then. Why should the baby feed at 9.30? Drift along with it all, for the short, sleepless, crazy months, and one day it will all settle. The best way to get a pattern is suddenly to notice, quite to your surprise, that the baby has been asking for feeds at roughly the same time each day for a week. Fancy that. What a coincidence. Can't possibly last ... and then it does last, and you have a settled baby, and can begin craftily to manipulate its meals to suit yourself.

Incidentally, it is not uncommon for these mad unpatterned weeks to take their toll of new mothers' nerves; plenty of women can't relax or sleep at all by day, simply because the baby *might* cry. Most of us have lain, tensely, in bed, or read the same newspaper headline ten times over, expecting every minute to hear a wail from the bedroom. You can waste a whole three-hour sleep of the baby's this way, and greet it again with tense irritability when it does wake. The best cure for the condition is not Valium, but to get someone else – anyone reasonably reliable will do – simply to take the baby *out of the house*, in a pram, round and round the block with a promise not to bring it back for at least an hour and a half. Your mother, father, husband, neighbour, any sensible sixteen-year-old can do this small thing for you; it may be a lifeline. It is no disgrace to ask for it.

Night and day ... you are the one ... who gets up to the baby. It is the one great disadvantage of breastfeeding. New babies don't know what night is for. They gradually find out because you become so much grumpier, quieter and less sociable after 10 p.m. Next to the problem of entertaining them through the day, the problem of getting some unbroken sleep is the greatest. Tough tactics only prolong the agony; your nerve will crack before the baby stops crying, and you might as well get up straight away. At first, some babies refuse to go back to sleep after a night feed, and this is desperate. But it does gradually improve: even persistent night-feeders lose that appalling habit after a few weeks, and drop quietly off with the feed over. And slowly, the night sleeps lengthen. Some people try to speed it up by tiring the baby out during the evening; some set up elaborate rituals of nightdresses and hair-brushing and singing and putting-to-bed in a special night-time cot in a special night-time room; one friend has a rocking cradle next to the bed, and lies half-asleep with one foot attached to the cradle bars with an old belt, rocking the baby. (There is, of course, no strictly biological reason why you can't fix the belt to your husband's foot and get him to do the twitching.) After four or five months, it is worth trying the old trick of offering only water at night; a lot of babies are bright enough to work out that water isn't worth waking up for.

But actually, if you stay cool, take advantage of every offer of help or short cut during the day, and expect nothing much of your very small offspring, it may actually happen that the baby tires of night-waking before you do. A mother of three said to me, 'You learn that it all goes so quickly. It seems that the ghastly bits go on forever, and suddenly they're grown up. I truly enjoyed night feeds with the youngest – it was so nice to have a little thing slurping away in the middle of the night, and I knew I wouldn't have for long.' I felt much the same with my own first child: I was doing a taxing job all day, and regretted his eight hours with the nanny, ten miles from my desk. The nights were a magical, private time when he smiled fatly on the changing-mat and gently stroked my breast. I used to have an Agatha Christie handy, and read for half an hour sometimes while he sucked, half-asleep. When I had finished all the Agatha Christies in the house, he was ten months old and the taxing job was ending. So I sent my husband in with a bottle of water for three nights running, and he gave up waking. It was the end of an era. To this day I can't pass a station bookstall display of Agatha Christies without feeling a milky tingling come over me ...

Clothes

This is the one area in which you can totally please yourself, if you think about it. Short of overheating, freezing or infestation with lice, there is not much you can do which the new baby will care tuppence about. There seem to be two schools of thought. One says, 'Put them in Babygros,

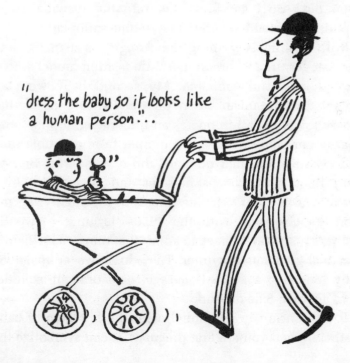

"dress the baby so it looks like a human person"...

things with hoods and feet, zip-up pram bags ['baby-cosies'], and to hell with boots, hats, buttons, straps and extras of all kinds.' The other says, 'dress the baby so that it looks like a human person and not like a towelling sausage. Persons are easier to put up with when they throw up, wake you etc. than are sausages.'

There is something to be said for this latter view, whatever hellish fumblings with designer dungarees it leads to: I put my first child into very snappy 'real' clothes from the start, and on the one occasion I fiddled him into a trad white cardigan and bonnet to please his Granny, my husband was quite upset. 'Oh God,' he blurted. 'He looks like a bloody *baby* or something.' (The lad was all of a fortnight old.) So I got him back into the Ipswich Town supporter striped hat and the navy-blue sailor suit.

Still, washing is washing and changing is changing, and you can get tired of dressing a little fashion-model whose clothes are a full-time job. My second baby wore an amiable compromise, based on the Babygro or similar dreary towelling all-in-one as an underlayer, topped with a jazzy tank-top or sleeveless jumper from a jumble sale, and possibly finished off with those wonderful Bierton Baby Boots with sheepskin soles and ankle ties which defeat pulling off. Having mocked repeatedly at my mother's obsession with the 1950s 'leggings' – woolly trousers with feet – I have to admit that they are brilliantly practical garments in winter. They do, however, make the baby look like a knitted sausage, or a draught-excluder from a parish Sale of Work.

It is a curiously emotional area, the business of baby clothes. When you are first pregnant, it can symbolize the

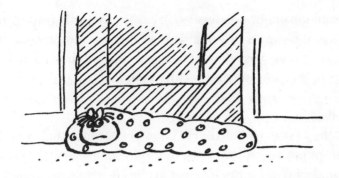

whole of the uncharted, unfamiliar ocean of parenthood: I used to wander for hours in department stores, gazing in terror at the different types of baby-vest – envelope-neck or crossover or bodysuit – and wondering how I would ever keep a child alive, let alone dressed. Now I become passionately evangelical about such technicalities as the bodysuit with poppers under the legs (the only thing which keeps inefficiently fixed nappies on) and the meanness of manufacturers who fail to extend the front zip down the inside of one leg (thus forcing you to bend the little beast's knee up, which he or she may not like one little bit). None of my friends is entirely agreed about the correct way to dress a baby (although it did not seem to stop us borrowing off one another with great abandon and sending sackfuls of moulting, tattered, outgrown clothes across the country between babies), so I will merely quote my sister-in-law on the subject. Her house is a kind of Crewe Junction of every kind of tiny garment, and her technique at jumble sales is the talk of Lincolnshire. 'Always say yes to everything that's offered,' she says. 'It may seem like rubbish, but will come in handy when everything is in the washing basket.' At such moments, arguments about persons vs. sausages dwindle into irrelevance. It seems a pity that it is also at such moments that long-lost relatives come to call, bringing all their friends to admire your ragged and scruffy baby ...

Habitats

The biggest waste of time I have ever committed was the brief phase when I thought that new babies – too small to lie and play on a rug and get grubby – actually needed to be put into nighties or pyjamas in the evening. After a bit, I saw the error of my ways, and didn't even put them in a separate container for the night. I evolved a very efficient 'containerization' system which would be the envy of many a cargo shipping company. The baby lived in a light Moses basket lined with a soft lambskin (the sort they sell for nursing premature babies, and which seems to make all babies happier to go to bed). At night, the basket fitted into the cradle by the bed; for travelling in the car, it fitted into an old rigid carrycot kept permanently strapped in the back seat. The rest of the time, the basket sat on the kitchen bench, or the sitting-room sofa, or wherever I happened to be. That way, I never had to disturb the baby at all, and it could do what infants most like to do, which is set its own pattern of sleeping and waking. If I had waited another couple of years there would have been an even better and much safer piece of equipment on the market: I reel with jealousy at the sheer convenience of those reclining seats which fit into a car seat-belt backwards (very safe) and then can be unceremoniously hoiked out and brought indoors, or to a cafe table or on to the beach. The only caveat there is that you shouldn't leave even a small baby in it all day and night: they need to lie down flat sometimes, just like we do. If you're not having to get in and out of cars during the day, that is one reason why an old-fashioned pram can be a godsend (especially with its shopping-tray at the bottom). But then you need a big hallway.

Organize the transport in a way that suits you, and you will never have to hover around wondering whether to wake the baby to go to the shops; you don't have to declare an official bedtime, waking the baby to shift it to its official cot. If you keep handy near the baby seat or basket or pram a couple of nappies, a tube of baby wipes, a spare Babygro and muslin square, and a tiny jar of zinc-and-castor-oil ointment, the baby is never without an instant change, and you don't have to miss half a television programme, stop a conversation, or climb an unnecessary flight of stairs in order to do everything it needs. Thinking your way through the system saves a lot of bad temper and minimizes the sense of being put-upon and constantly interrupted.

There are endless peculiar variations on this theme of portable habitats: one friend of mine with long strong arms eccentrically carried her child around the house in a baby-bath, claiming that it was wonderfully light and draught proof, and that the lambskin made it warm as well. Another had a cardboard box in every room with a firm cushion in it, covered in an old pillowcase, and moved the baby around in a cocoon with handles ('only there had been warnings about *smothering* in cocoons, so I had to keep looking'). Another went everywhere, and did every job, with her baby asleep or awake in a sling; but she used to be a gymnast, and had amazing back and neck muscles. Once the baby gets to the propping-up stage, you can have a very light lean-back chair or bouncing-cradle in every part of the house, if you keep remorselessly borrowing them from all your friends as soon as their babies learn to sit alone; the phase is so short that a moderate-sized network of friends is likely to have at least three redundant lean-back chairs at any one time. All in all, the practice of endlessly 'popping up to the nursery' to check on the baby or change its nappy is best left where it belongs, in very old-fashioned TV situation comedies.

Incidentally, all the nursery shops will try to sell you a 'changing chest', with diddy little shelves and a fold-out top for changing the baby on 'without back strain'. I know a few mothers who swear by these, but don't be too downcast if you can't raise the money. I didn't buy one because I couldn't raise the *nerve;* I knew, deep down inside me, that one day I would do the banned, dangerous thing and turn away for a moment from the baby on the very day it learned to roll. Crash. Horror. A four-foot drop. On the other hand, changing-mats on the floor really do strain your back after a while; so I got a great big old hamper, filled it with spare blankets, and put a plastic mat on it. In our house, we changed babies by sinking to our knees beside the hamper. Neither ever rolled off, as it happens, but if they had, the fall would have been a short one.

Travelling
There are several good reasons for getting around as much as possible with a new baby. One is that staying at home with it can be so terrible; another is that when the baby

gets a bit bigger, travelling will be harder, the child that much heavier, and your expedition less warmly welcomed. Everybody likes to meet a nice little bundle sucking at the breast or dozing in a basket; but a roving, grabbing, food-throwing vandal will lose you friends. Especially if he or she is at that delicate stage when one disruption to the daily routine means hours of whining and a hysterical refusal to go to bed. Infants have no routine, no preconceptions, and only want to be where you, the milk, and the lambskin basket are. Take advantage. Another good reason for taking holidays, visiting distant relations, or even (as I did) travelling wildly all over the place on jobs, is that the more sociable a baby's first few months are, the better it seems to take to strangers later. Apart from a few brief bouts of clinging, both of mine got remarkably social, due (I like to think) to their early savoir-faire picked up in BBC lifts, railway carriages, aeroplanes, motorway cafes and everybody else's house.

One warning, though: a competent and contented new mother once embarked on her first social outing with her new baby, dressing herself up carefully for the first time since the birth, and finishing off with a dab of her favourite scent – again for the first time since the birth. She tenderly picked the baby up for his feed when she reached her friend's house, proud to show off her expertise at breastfeeding and the placidity of her son – and he screamed in terror, arching away from her, refusing to suck and generally behaving like a vampire confronted with a crucifix. *He didn't like the perfume.* Once she had realized, and washed it off while the baby howled on her friend's lap, he was perfectly all right again.

Transport

Cars are all very well, but can run you ragged with nerves when the infant starts to grizzle on the motorway or in a traffic-jam. I once drove from Suffolk to Manchester and back in a weekend, however, without one cross noise from the back. What I had done was to sling a cradle toy with rattling bits and pieces above the three-month-old baby's carrycot, anchoring one end to the handle of the petrol-can in the boot, and the other to the headrest of the driver's seat. Whenever she woke up, I fed and changed her in a lay-by ('No, no, officer, no problems with the car, just the sticky-tape on this nappy, you wouldn't have a roll of Sellotape in that tool bag, would you?') and laid her on her back to watch the jangly plastic cymbals. The only disadvantage to the system came days later, when I ran out of petrol on the way home for a feed and had to sprint down to the local garage carrying baby on one arm and on the other the petrol-can, which was pathetically adorned with a stringful of plastic bells and rings, too intricately tied to get off in a hurry. Still, mothers get used to funny looks from passers-by.

Public transport is daunting. 'Nothing', says one mother I questioned, 'makes one feel more desperate and victimized.' 'You must be *quite forceful* about demanding help from the public and co-operation from bus conductors,' said another, grimly. 'Just don't go,' said no fewer than 21 others. All this is true enough, if you stick to short-term journeys, the urban bus being possibly the worst environment ever devised for a mother and baby; but that shouldn't put anybody off doing longer journeys.

Trains are perfect, especially half-empty long-distance ones with big tables to put the carrycot down on. Nicholas did two thousand miles or so by rail before he was six months old, and a dozen flights; and Rose travelled from East Suffolk to central London once or twice a week for six months. There was no element of self-sacrifice or Perfect Motherhood in this: I just happen to enjoy myself more, in the first six months, when I know exactly where the baby is and exactly what it is doing. I tried the other way – leaving bottles of breast milk and sprinting to get back for the next feed – and found it much more peaceful jiggling the miles away with the baby perched half-propped in the basket, gazing out at the passing scenery and digesting its feed, while I listened to my Walkman, read a paper, and ate a sandwich. When I arrived ready to do the job at the other end, I would hand the baby over to a nurse from a local agency, booked in advance, for the few hours the job actually took. No baby is likely to come to any harm in three hours with a trained nurse, and its mother half a mile away on the end of the telephone.

To manage long journeys, though (or short ones), you need to have a totally professional approach. Expect absolutely nothing to be on tap; ignore all airline propaganda about 'sky-cots' and bottle-warmers, and never trust even the lushest train to have so much as a beaker of hot water. Pack a great clanking bagful of everything, including a little waterproof mat to change the baby on, and hang the bag from your shoulder on a stout strap. Do not ignore your own needs: I once considerably startled a departure lounge at Heathrow by bending tenderly over my wicker baby-basket, smoothing the sleeping infant's hair, and hauling out from under the blanket by his feet a can of Guinness stout and a Cornish pasty.

When packing, on no account omit the Squeaky Duck
(if the baby is over a month or so). Nothing alleviates boredom quite like a nice squeaky duck between the jaws.
Munch, munch, squeak, squeak. Once, after a dawn journey from Lincolnshire to London, I handed the baby to his
father, and rushed out to lunch with the new editor of the
Tatler at the Gay Hussar restaurant. Very fashionable, very
literary. It was not really the place to delve in one's handbag, hit the abandoned rubber duck by accident, and
deafen the diners with a muffled but resounding squeak.
Lord Longford, at the next table, froze with his fork
halfway to his mouth …

The other useful tactic for baby-laden travellers is to get
on your plane or into your carriage, and stroll down the
aisle, brandishing a sweet little chubby face from side to
side until you hear the magic syllable, 'Aaaah!' Then sit
down, as close to the 'Aaaah' as possible, and you have
found yourself a baby-freak prepared to work hard for a
smile the whole journey long. Generally, elderly ladies or
schoolgirls are the best bet; but not always. One of the
greatest successes ever was a severe-looking EEC engineer-
ing consultant on his way to Newcastle, who not only
wiggled his ears and made a rattle out of a crushed beer
can, but eagerly permitted Nicholas to chew up a whole
edition of *Chartered Mechanical Engineer* magazine.

Another thing which I find helpful is to keep the frills
and the helplessness down. Even a well-fed, amused,
urbane and cheerful baby can be met with cold, horrified
stares in some carriages and aeroplanes. Businessmen may
just have left a home full of yowling children, and be looking forward to some quiet work; businesswomen may have

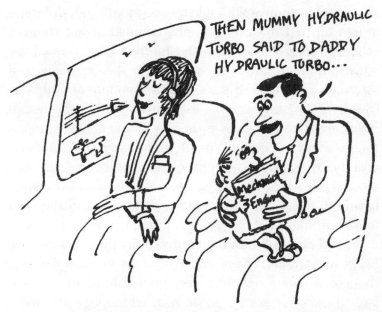

left their own babies, rather sadly, with nannies. So an infant in a plain jumpsuit with an efficient-looking mother is going to be less irritating, and attract more helpful hands, than some apparition in a beribboned white lace bassinet, attended by a chaotic tearful milkmaid of a Mum dropping bottles and bootees everywhere. If you refrain from brandishing disturbing bits of nursery gear at sour-looking bachelors with Britoil clipboards, and don't shower their annual accounts with talcum powder and dribble, you are more likely to get helped off the train the other end with a civil word. Even, perhaps, praised for your baby's behaviour.

But rely on no help; Outlaw Mum, alone on the trail, should never take anything she can't carry alone. And don't assume even basic intelligence in anybody. I got

aboard a plane once with a baby one month old; the stew-
ardess bustled towards me, programmed at her training
school to Help Travellers with Children. She assessed the
situation, then tittupped off on her 4-inch heels and
returned with the airline's official version of Help for
Children: a jigsaw puzzle. I explained, gently, that the lad
didn't even *chew* jigsaw puzzles yet; she almost grasped
the idea, but not quite. When I began, very discreetly and
cleanly, to change his nappy on the empty seat between
me and the window (yes, yes, on a rubber mat) her contri-
bution to the welfare of young travellers was to suggest I
took him, in mid-change, to the minute lavatory compart-
ment and changed him on its tiny, filthy floor. No chance,
I said sweetly, and she flounced off. I am not complaining,
though; we were having a very enjoyable flight. We just
had to grow an extra skin or two, which was not much
trouble. Not with all that nice airline gin inside us.

However, travels with a new baby, however careful you
are and however cool, can turn out dreadfully. I never
have smugly congratulated myself on my expertise; rather,
at the end of every trip, I said, 'Well, we got away with
that one.' It is probably easier for working-travelling mothers like me, who get used to every awkwardness and learn
to judge to a hair's breadth whether the carrycot can be
wedged on the next seat in the dining-car while we eat
breakfast; but even with every sort of experience you can
come unstuck.

I once spent three and a half terrible hours on a train,
going to a television programme. In the seats opposite
were my fellow-guests, the most unkind and anti-baby
gossip journalist in London, and a mildly effete, definitely

babyless Leader of Cafe Society. There was nowhere else on the train to move to; I, and they, were stuck. The child grizzled uncharacteristically for the entire trip; fed incessantly, and filled countless appallingly scented nappies, which I had to creep to the lavatory to change. I ran out of clean plastic bags. Anticipating crucifixion, public and private, at the hands of the smooth and sneering devils opposite, I grew gloomier and gloomier and the baby crosser and crosser. Just outside Newcastle, he finally fell asleep; and as his mouth fell open a little I spied a miracle.

'Oh look!' I cried, forgetting my unsympathetic company. 'He's got a TOOTH!'

Suddenly, everyone was fascinated.

'Gosh!' said the socialite. 'Do they come just, er, like that?'

'Oh, I remember my daughter's first tooth,' burbled the unkind old gossip-writer, suddenly transformed like Ebenezer Scrooge. 'Wonderful, isn't it? But you'll never see that toothless grin again!'

And we all pulled up at the station beaming triumphantly, united by the little bit of ivory. Infants have a way of redeeming themselves in the nick of time. Just as well, really.

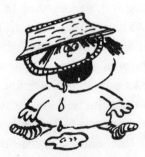

• •

Chapter Four

From Bundle to Vandal: Bigger Babies

We used to have a rota at the weekends with our first baby. At set intervals the cry would ring out, 'I've had him since 9.35, you take him till 12.00.' You can see families on holiday, in restaurants, making even shorter deals:

'Look, I've had her on my knee for seven minutes, so it's someone else's turn, we said five each.'

'Yes, but you had the carrot-sticks to give her, Sue and Brian had to manage her during the soup, that's not fair.'

'Oh, all right then, but it's Mum's turn again in a minute, think she's getting tired of my knee anyway, she doesn't seem to want to bang the salt-cellar any more.'

It isn't that nobody loves the baby – if they didn't, they wouldn't have brought it, or be trying to keep it happy – it is just the total, exhausting concentration caused by a questioning mind, increasingly agile hands, and a total lack of restraint. Parents at certain stages of babyhood feel hopeless. The books say that the baby needs toys – but they never mention that he will get through them with the ruthless speed and contempt of a newspaper editor spiking stories about lost cats. Educational posting-boxes,

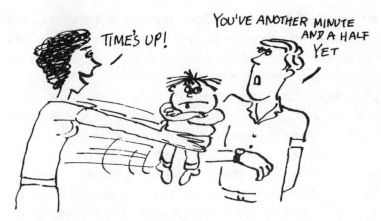

beautiful wooden trains, wobbly caterpillars, roly balls –
all examined, discarded and forgotten in minutes. It is
almost as if the baby was looking for something – the ulti-
mate egg-box, perhaps, or some particularly fine serving-
spoon reputed to be buried beyond the Mountains of the
Moon.

Then the books say that the baby needs to be played
with and 'stimulated' by adult company. So you do peek-
a-boo, you do this-is-the-way-the-farmer-rides, you try to
show him how to put a brick in a square hole. Each diversion lasts three minutes. But he is awake ten or twelve
hours a day ... you panic. He has thrown away all the toys
and everything in the kitchen. Suddenly, he finds a roll of
lavatory paper, and becomes hopelessly engrossed. He
doesn't want you to play with him. Doesn't notice if you
leave the room, even. Defeated, you slink off to finish the
washing-up, until a furious cry from the floor behind you
tells you that the roll of paper has abruptly lost its charm.

For a spell, we lived in a highly inappropriate new
house (unsafe concrete floor in the most used room, the

kitchen, and the only safe floor upstairs, in a playroom too far from adult occupations). We felt as if we were nothing but a pair of ever-vigilant security guards, there to prevent disaster and escape, but not particularly welcomed as playmates. All the boy wanted to do was explore, with passion and concentration, everything available; then loudly shriek for new worlds to conquer. It was a dark, wet, freezing winter, in the depths of the country with neighbours yet to be met; in short, it was a pretty low ebb. But the tide always rises again, with babies; nothing lasts; the most unreasonable, nightmarish phases melt away overnight.

I remember asking my mother, a little earlier than that wintry Colditz era – probably when my son was about nine months old – how long it was, generally, before you could put a baby down on a double bed for a moment and be fairly sure that he wouldn't crawl straight off and land on his head. 'Oh,' she said confidently, 'not until about three years old. You have to watch them every single minute, for years.' Whereupon I gave serious consideration to throwing myself on my own head, out of the nearest window. Luckily, though, she was wrong. All mothers suffer from selective amnesia: the long tunnel of babyhood is remembered only in brief, impressionistic flashes which obscure all sorts of little developments and welcome changes. In retrospect, you forget those great intellectual leaps by the baby which change its parents' lives overnight. The classic one, for us, was when Nicholas finally understood the command, 'NOT IN YOUR MOUTH!' He was about eleven months old. Suddenly, the number of things he could be allowed to play with was quadrupled – plasticine, coal, candles, sand, pebbles, potatoes crusted with earth. It was wonderful. For us, that is: it ushered in a new age of distractibility and peace. Within a week, it seemed incredible that there had ever been a time when we could not lie serenely in bed of a morning, drinking tea, with a small rapt figure between us gazing in adoration at a paraffin candle which he had longed to hold for weeks, but would have chewed before. As for the crawling-off-the-bed problem, what my mother should have remembered is the gradual process by which the baby stares over the edge, throws a few toys over, has a minor bump himself, and puts two and two together. Slowly, it becomes less and less likely that he will fall off things, except entirely by accident; when he gets nimbler all round, accidents themselves become fewer. There is not a lot you can do to speed up all these changes; given reasonable freedom to pull himself around, explore, and meet new people and new objects, a normal baby gets on very nicely with the job of developing. I was reduced almost to tears once by a reproving perfectionist of a mother who – when I asked if there were any short cuts – replied sternly: 'There are no short cuts in child development or mothering skills.' Phooey. The short cut is to love the baby, keep it from actual harm, cart it about with you, feed it, give it plenty of things to bang, and to hell with educational psychology, Infant Massage, or waving flash-cards at it all day. It is magical to watch things happening by themselves (and life, incidentally, becoming easier for you). You put furniture away, rightly fearing that your low coffee-table is a deathtrap for your laboriously wobbly, newly pulling-up baby – but in three months' time, you suddenly realize that the baby is inches taller, and gets up without pulling on anything anyway. Back comes the little table. You worry for weeks about how to stop a tricycling child crashing over the step in the hall, leaping on him ten times an hour, but by the time you have designed a set of ramps and gates, he has worked out the danger for himself and stopped going near it. No sooner do you perfect your arrangement of lean-back chairs in every key room than the baby sits up straight, wobbling triumphantly, on its little fundament. You puree every meal, out of habit, and get spoon-feeding down to a fine art; then one day you take the baby out to tea and when nobody is watching, she does a boarding-house-reach across the table, pinches a cucumber sandwich and eats it whole and unaided. You install stair-gates, and eight months later you hardly ever use them. It all happens very gradually, and total amnesia sets in afterwards. In retrospect it is all pretty easy, and parents all behave like those people who come home from

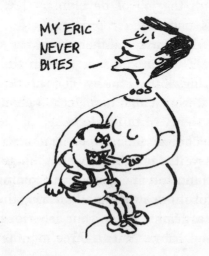

MY ERIC
NEVER
BITES —

holiday saying, 'Never a drop of rain!' when it actually lashed down for two days.

What this means is that much general advice is unhelpful, and that a visit from a friend with a slightly older (or slightly different) baby can plunge you into gloom at your own ineptitude.

'Oh,' they trill, 'we never had any trouble with Jasmine and light-plugs, she's always been very sensible. We just say "No" and she understands perfectly ... Oh, Eric knows that his bed is for sleeping – he goes straight off, always has ...' Or: 'The thing about safety is to be *quite firm* from the start. Samantha has always been told that the fire is hot, so of course she keeps away from it! It's a question of your approach.'

These mothers have no idea that they are lying through their teeth: they have just forgotten, as we all mercifully forget, that Jasmine spent three weeks laying siege to every light-fitting in the house, that Eric shrieked and rattled the cot-bars every evening until a fortnight ago, and that Samantha was never safe for two minutes in any room with a fire until last spring; and that since then, there have been three months of hot summer, and she has grown up enough to be told. Or it could be (evil thought) that Jasmine is a bit behindhand and hasn't actually noticed the wall-fittings yet ... she will, she will.

Sometimes the books and advisers forget, too, and move rapidly on from rattles and cot-mobiles to suggestions that you make caterpillars out of egg-boxes. Save your energy. There is a long phase during which the baby would just as soon have the egg-box. Imagination, pretending, all the mental handles which enable a toddler to be kept amused with a pair of cotton reels and a stick, have not developed in this big, mobile, enquiring baby. He is literal-minded: what he wants is the egg-box. Once that has been sucked, thrown, squashed and waved in the air (two and a half minutes approximately) he wants the wooden spoon. And the garlic-press. And the car-keys. And the rolling-pin. And the breadknife, the meat-skewers and the bottle of bleach. Frankly, if he can't have them, you ought to have put them somewhere he can't see; it saves time, in the end. We had a box of spoons and utensils on the wall, and every time you carried a baby past it he or she had to have something. Once, the box conveniently included the sharp tin-opener, the edgy fish-slice and the glass rolling-pin. Not for long, it didn't.

During all this year of transition from dear little bundle to storm-trooping vandal, the baby overreaches itself. You start to notice, in the immobile days, that the infant who can only gaze is wobbling his hand; wants to swipe. The swiper wants to grab, the grabber endlessly practises letting go (over the edge of the pram, as a rule). The floppy baby may not have developed his back muscles, but still lunges forward, wanting to sit up; the sitter wants to stand; the immobile wants to get on the move, and develops extraordinary bottom-shuffling, seal-humping, rolling and bouncing ways of dragging round the room. (My daughter had a most peculiar system, rather like a man in a cartoon heaving himself over the sand to an oasis – all elbows and forearms.) On a good day, this overreaching gives them hours of entertainment. On bad days, they keep falling over and getting stuck under things and shrieking vengeance and damnation on the universe, and you can't so much as mash a potato without stopping at least twice to rescue them. Then your mother-in-law drops in to observe that pulling up too early to their feet 'makes babies' legs grow up bandy'.

On the good days, you pose like an illustration in a motherhood magazine, thoughtfully handing your child a clean, educational rattle from time to time and exchanging polite 'Ah goos' to develop his Social Skills. On a bad day you observe bitterly, across the sea of crumpled and chewed rubbish, that every new skill the baby develops means more trouble. I spent fond, proud hours teaching my son to work his toy nut-and-bolt from the Early Learning Centre, screwing the plastic nut off and on again. Days later, screw-top lids began mysteriously coming off everything, and I had to stop letting him play with the shampoo bottles in the bath. You teach him to pile bricks, thinking he will be the new Brunel; next thing you know, jam-jars are crashing everywhere from a NatWest glass tower brilliantly constructed on the breakfast-table. Play therapeutic 'pouring' games in the bath, as recommended by child psychologists, and equally therapeutic pouring will flood the highchair with warm milk three times a day.

Another source of confusion is that a growing baby actually needs a different mother from the one who suited the newborn so well. The new, crazily unpatterned, impulsive baby needs a sort of laid-back, faintly hippie mother – perfectly happy to go to bed at 1 a.m., to have lunch at different times three days running, never know what the time is or have any outside appointments. She generally drifts along with the newborn eccentric, taking life as it comes.

Then, at a certain stage (which nobody can quite pin down, but which seems to happen somewhere between the first tooth and the first crawl), this free-floating mother has to become a military-routine freak, always ready to slap lunch down on the dot of 12.15, get the baby in bed for a nap at 1.00 precisely, or whatever. All the things which were crazy when nurses or in-laws suggested them for newborns (strict routine, definite mealtimes, pyjamas at night) suddenly become useful for the bigger baby. This no doubt explains why the advisers kept pushing them in the first place – a touch of maternal amnesia and selective memory – but it is dreadfully confusing. When my first baby was 11 months old I wanted to take him to a local toddler group, but it ran from 10.00 until 12.00. I dithered around helplessly for a while saying, 'Well, he generally seems to want his morning sleep sometime between 9.30 and 11 o'clock' as if he was an unpredictable month-old blob in a basket. Then suddenly one day I had had enough, and decided to take an initiative myself. The nap was officially moved to one o'clock; and after two days of keeping him up all morning and putting him down after lunch, he settled into a pattern which endured for two years. The sense of power was heady. So Baby No. 2 was under martial law as soon as she was six months old.

The snag about routines is that although it is delightful when the baby sticks to them, waking up at a time you can handle, taking a predictable nap, having a proper bedtime, you have to stick to them too. Once the baby gets used to the idea that it can skip the after-lunch nap, get overtired, whinge all afternoon, drop off to sleep at 5.30 too tired to eat supper, wake up hungry at 10.00, sit up with Mummy and Daddy until midnight and fall asleep in their bed, that is the kind of life you are locking yourself into, and may God have mercy on your soul. One or two days don't seem to matter; a week or a fortnight does.

Dozens of people say things like, 'Oh, he was having a daytime nap until we went on holiday and he got out of the habit,' or, 'He slept in his cot until we stayed at Granny's and he got to like a bed.' This is fine, as long as the change is one you wanted. Myself, I have gone to ridiculous lengths to prevent the ruin of a routine which suited me, the family, the baby and got the day finished in good order. I bullied Sunday lunch guests into getting here in time to eat at 1.00 sharp; I took sheepskins and folding cots out to lunch so the children could be tucked away as usual to sleep it off; I observed, for a period, the bath-play-story-bed routine at 7.00 each evening with the fanaticism of an Ayatollah. People who say babies ought to be free to express their individual needs about bedtime, naps, etc. are welcome to take the consequences. In the ten hours a day that they are awake and at large, most of the ones I know express quite enough individuality to be getting on with ...

The nice thing about this stage, between floppy, baffling infancy and rebellious two-year-old, is that the whole business of childcare can be demystified. Looking after a new baby, you have to listen to a few experts, you have to read a book or two: things have to be sterilized, heads supported, nappies anxiously peered into. An alien has landed. Six months later, the business of nappies and diet is more or less automatic, the baby feels firm and strong when you pick it up, joins in smiles and jokes, and likes

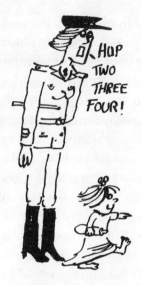

sitting at meals with everyone else. The most reluctant
fathers tend to fall in love at this stage, and strangers
consent to having their glasses ripped off by your beaming, charming, cuddly little friend. You know the baby's
foibles (like terror of ripping Velcro, or a passion for
bananas). It becomes much harder for anybody to make
you feel guilty or inadequate, when the baby is so trans-
parently cheerful, banging its spoon on the table or shouting incomprehensible oaths at the cat.

On the other hand, Competition rears its dreadful head.
Although it should be perfectly clear to everyone that your
child is exceptionally intelligent, beautiful and sweet-
natured, other mothers are remarkably obtuse about this.
As Pam Ayres immortally put it:

> '... it's hard to explain, when I look at your Wayne,
> Why *you* bothered to have one at all!'

Other babies sit up sooner than yours (but not so charm-ingly). They are alleged to say 'Da-da' at eight months. They have more hair (well, so do chimpanzees). They sleep longer, walk sooner, and may even be held out over potties at a year old. All this is quite bearable, as long as they are babies you know personally, have round for tea sometimes, and can silently criticize to yourself by way of consolation. It is quite *un*bearable when parents of older children, or grandparents, start making wild, crazy claims about their own historic offspring. Put cotton wool in your ears.

There is no shortage of instruction on how to look after babies, or amuse them; but specifically for this roving, grabbing, butterfly-minded stage, I have collected a few pearls from the more relaxed-looking of my acquaintance. Some of them may sound crazy, mildly unhygienic, impossible or psychologically dubious, but that is one of the joys of motherhood: criticizing other mothers for their peculiar systems, then surreptitiously stealing a few.

Amusements
The great knack is never expecting them to last very long. Babies need to be kept busy, like troublemaking peasants in the Middle Ages being set to dig pointless ditches by their cunning overlord. At the first whimper from the playpen, pounce, whip infant out, and put it in the bouncer, or the highchair with a toy, or whatever else you have as an alternative. Always have your pocket full of surprises, cotton reels, balloons or bubble tubs when you go out. (I used to draw large crowds of older children on station platforms as I blew bubbles for a pushchair baby.)

Anticipate boredom all the time: hang rattly toys in the car, by the baby-seat. Keep a few unpainted wooden curtain-rings (eyelets removed) round the handles of the buggy for chewing. Some tried and tested and very cheap favourite games at home are:

- Magazine shredding. This is made much cheaper by the kindness of commercial firms who push junky catalogues through the door. Newspapers are also handy, although someone once told me that the only non-poisonous newsprint in Britain is the *Financial Times*. I have never been able to check this.
- Soapflake Alley was the name of a splendid tunnel of boxes taped together for the babies to crawl through, built by a father I know. It lasted ages, on their bedroom floor, enabling them to lie in bed longer in the morning while their boys crawled through avenues of old soap, TV and microwave cartons from the shop down the road. Check the boxes for sharp staples, though.
- The saucepan cupboard. King of them all; every single mother I know says that her baby emptied the saucepan cupboard daily for months. It is so common that I would not even mention it, except that I want to tell you that once a month you should check the size of all the pans (and cake-rings – especially cake-rings, my God) to make sure that none of them has become that exact size which the baby can jam on to its head and not get off. If you don't and the worst happens, remember that a thin aluminium pan or cake-ring can be gently bent, and that a baby's head is actually oval,

front-to-back; you can sometimes squeeze gently over the ears and win enough space to slide it off the brow. Baby-oil helps. A bit.

- Messing. Lentils, water, sand, flour, rice and avert your eyes from the result. Painting is similarly chaotic, but the great knack is to persuade granny/daddy/nanny/minder that their creative talents and artistic flair mean that they, and they alone, are fit to teach your one-year-old to paint while you do something more soothing, like washing the car or peeling potatoes.

- Girls. If you can capture a girl between nine and thirteen, the odds are that you have a totally dedicated, patient, inventive baby-amuser for the afternoon. A few boys are as good but (sorry, feminists) they tend to be a bit more frightening and less gentle.

- Visitors. Fill the house with people. Have the rewiring or plumbing done. Invite firms round to estimate for double-glazing. Have dissolute and feckless bachelor uncles to stay on the sofa overnight. Nothing is worse than to be stuck, eyeball-to-eyeball, with a lone baby all day; you get sick of each other. Any outside company is better than none. I struck a bargain with my large, then childless extended family: I would feed huge numbers for Sunday lunch, provided that at least two turn up at 10.30 to keep the babies amused. At Christmas we went further, and had an official Duty Uncle who had to be there at 8.30 to jolly-up the children while we cooked.

- Unpacking. It is actually worth packing a small suitcase specifically so that the baby can unpack it all over the floor. If the baby can't open them yet, a good wheeze is to put in unopened bags of crisps or crinkly sweet-bags, hidden among the folds of shawls and scarves. A quick pack-up in the evening can enable you to lie in bed drinking tea for a full half-hour while the baby fossicks around happily.

- Books. Amazingly popular, amazingly early. If you value your sanity, don't buy ones with irritating stories. They are bound to turn into favourites later, and after a particularly stressful period, I decided that if I had to read *Polly Pig and the Bee* once more, I would emigrate.

- Kitchen sink. Fill it with warm water. Take the baby's clothes off. Put the baby in the sink with a few plastic mugs. Potter nearby, keeping a watchful eye. This is a brilliant way to get the ironing done without interference.

- Bird table. Endless free entertainment. If you're lucky, a cat will climb up as well, and keep falling off. Flat-dwellers note the RSPB stick-on bird table which fixes to a windowpane with suckers: it comes by mail order.

- Food. While you cannot stuff them full of snacks to shut them up all the time, you can resort to a wonderful substance called 'Tropical Mix' – dried fruits, shards of coconut etc. – because a small handful contains very few calories and takes ages to eat. Get the kind without chokey, allergy-producing peanuts, though. You can also claim to be encouraging pincer action and manual dexterity, if any of your Build-A-Better-Baby friends walk in.

- Music. Surprisingly cheering and soothing, again surprisingly early. My son's first word was 'Reggae Reggae'.

- Megaphones. This one sounds very silly, but it worked on my daughter for months. When the baby is sitting in the playpen shouting with boredom, get something like a big cardboard tube from a whisky-bottle, or the large inside of a kitchen-paper roll, or a light megaphone if you have one – and hold it in front of the shouting, crying face. The baby gets fascinated by the difference in its voice through the tube, and may well spend the next half-hour happily hooting into it.
- Mummy lying down. In moments of exhaustion when you feel you really ought to be 'playing with the baby', and he feels the same way, just lie down on the floor on your stomach (with a paperback if you like) and allow the infant to crawl all over you, climbing and rolling and giggling. Great pleasure for infant, minimal trouble for Mummy: altogether my kind of game. It survived, with the first child, well beyond the third birthday, since he could pretend I was a wrecked locomotive, and go round tapping my wheels with a foam-rubber hammer. The baby pretended I was a horse. I, meanwhile, could pretend to be on a beach in Corfu. All three of us were happy.

Finally, once a baby gets to eight or nine months old, the best way to get it interested in something is to play with the object yourself, in an absorbed fashion, for a few minutes. Then give it up, with a slight show of reluctance (this principle intensifies as time goes on, until the only way to get a toddler to wear its hat is to wear it for an hour yourself, without comment, before you go out). But if a baby does want something which you had no intention of giving it, stop for a moment and think hard before refusing. People who expect babies to play only with 'toys' are doomed to years of frustration and conflict. Why shouldn't he have the bicycle pump? The end of a hosepipe? A rubber torch? The Sellotape? A thick, heavy cosmetic jar he can't break? The Hoover? (One of ours used to stand just holding the handle, in a dreamlike respectful way, for half an hour at a time.) Or your old handbag? And why shouldn't he sit in a suitcase all day? The more things you refuse, the more ill-will and aggravation will build up between you. The trick is not to let him even *see* too many forbidden things; or at least, not see that they are portable.

Every year there are stories in the papers, headed 'OH, BABY!' or 'THE TERROR TOT!' They are about small children who by their first birthday have (there are always lots of stars and screamers in these stories):

★ SMASHED the stereo!
★ FLOODED the bathroom, ruining valuable furnishings!
★ COST Dad £500 in redecorating walls!
★ SCRATCHED a £5000 car! etc.

The parents, interviewed, proudly claim, 'He must be the naughtiest boy in the country! We don't know where to turn! He's cost us thousands!' It is all their own daft fault. Anyone with pencils accessible near good wallpaper, vases of flowers balanced on stereos, open bathroom doors or other insane invitations to mayhem is just too innocent to have a baby. You have to expect the very, very worst. All the time.

Bathtime
The best thing we ever found to bath a baby in at the just-sitting stage was a large builder's bucket. Supports the back and gives a great sense of security, with room to splash. Ours was on a boat, but you could put one inside the bath if you want to save hot water. At home, the main thing about bathtime is that you have to stay very close; so the knack is to make it a watery playpen while you sit and do something soothing, like paint your nails or wash your own hair. Myself, I read *Rumpole of the Bailey* short stories and played with the toy ducks.

Mealtime
Some spread newspaper or plastic under the highchair, but I prefer cleaning things I am fond of, like the house or the babies, to cleaning disgusting pieces of plastic. One friend carries this principle to extremes, says that she likes washing her children because she loves them, but hates washing clothes and nasty slimy bibs, so she feeds them supper naked, sometimes in the bath. A good hungry dog mooching around under the highchair helps.

As to food, babies get into the idea of finger-food much earlier than you think. After a few spoonfuls of nourishing baby-slime to assuage my conscience, mine just browsed from six months onwards on an assortment of toasted cheese, bread and honey, cooked peas, cucumber sandwiches, carrot, apple, celery, salami (in moderation), cold fish fingers, sausages, saltless crisps, wholewheat pasta shapes, avocado, Marmite fingers and toast.

Warmest votes for helpfulness, from my 50 mothers who filled in questionnaires, went to microwave ovens.

'Microwave to liquidizer to freeze to microwave to baby,' wrote one, tersely. And it does not need wealth. 'I paid for my microwave by doing relief petrol pumps while Carla slept in the car when she was tiny,' recalls one friend. 'Then I took a lodger for a few months to pay for my dishwasher.' Certainly anything which makes cooking proper food for a baby less of a bore and a chore is going to help; not least because it makes you less angry when he won't eat the stuff. If you let a neurotic fight about eating start now, you might have it for years. Just top hunger-strikers up with a mug of warm milk at bedtime and issue vitamin drops, hoping for the best.

Spoons are an issue. Some babies get into a spoon-grabbing habit long before they are actually fit to feed themselves. Rose had a system of grabbing one spoon, whereon I gave her the next spoonful out of another, and she grabbed that; so I picked up a third spoon, thinking that with both hands full she had no further power to grab. Whereon she would drop spoon no. 1, snatch spoon no.3 ... that is how the finger-food began.

What I should have done, according to a crafty old nanny, is to put bits of bread in both her hands, which she would be less likely to drop. Next time, I shall know. But the important thing to remember is that eventually the slowest baby will learn to use a spoon. If it amuses you to let him try early, it might be that he will be quite efficient, in a plastery sort of way, by nine months old. If you can't face the mess, that doesn't particularly matter either; just keep on spooning it in yourself.

Unfortunately, the single most useful thing to have at this stage is beyond your control: a totally bald baby is much easier to clean up than a well-thatched one.

Sunday afternoon

I put this in as a separate category just in order to pass on a wonderful idea practised by Chris Serle, his wife Anna and their baby Harry. They had Sunday tea in the playpen, in front of the fire. Chris and Anna sat in the playpen with all the Sunday papers, toasting crumpets through the bars. Harry had the run of the rest of the room, safe from the fire and unable to get at the papers.

Bedtime

This is the single greatest achievement of the first year. Nothing makes life more bearable than a baby who is happy to go to his cot in the evening, and stay there. It is worth a lot of trouble to establish this state of affairs, and escape the terrible circle of crying, waiting, rushing upstairs, upsetting the baby even more, coming down, listening for the next cry … Whether you have one of these bedtime devils to start with, or not, seems to be a matter of pure luck. My first child tormented us for a year, so much that we hardly dared leave him, even with his familiar daily nanny, after one night when he screamed so hard that even she – with years of experience – was driven to dash over the road with him to the neighbour for support. (Incidentally, he calmed down instantly he was out of the house. Babies are very receptive to a change of atmosphere, even a drizzling street, when they have filled a whole house with panicky vibrations of their own.) Ordinary babysitters were out of the question; we were filled with envy for friends who seemed to dump their six-month-olds with schoolgirls and go to the cinema without a backward glance. We thought we must be doing something terribly wrong.

Then the second child arrived, looked around, and promptly fell into a sleep from which she barely woke for two months except to feed. After night-feeding was over, she settled amiably in her cot every time, with barely a whimper, and woke smiling and still quite contented to lie and suck her muslin rag for an hour. Suddenly I understood that all those carefree, smug parents had not been geniuses after all – merely lucky first time round. Heaven help them if they get their evening-screamer next.

Families afflicted with bad bedtimes are irritable; and particularly irritated by advice, all of which they have tried. Warily, therefore, and with advance apologies, I would just pass on a few observations:

• Some babies are maddened by being rocked. If your baby dislikes it, don't assume you're doing it wrong, just stop. The same goes for tight swaddling, tucking-in and lullabies. If a cot is safe and a room is warm enough, there is no point interfering with whatever weird position the baby chooses to sleep in, even if it does the splits, or piles up all the blankets under its tummy. Once a baby is old enough to roll over, you can't stay neurotic about the safety 'Back to sleep position', or you'll go crazy trying to police it. Take nursery advice of the old school with a pinch of salt; it is only 60 years since mothers used to creep into their babies' rooms to tie up their little jaws with cloths and prevent them becoming Mouth Breathers.

• Colour psychologists say that pale or neutral colours really do help a baby to relax. I merely pass this on. I did once, in desperation, try draping a pale pink scarf

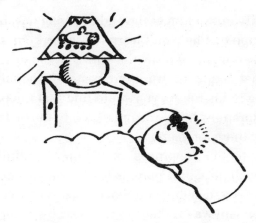

over the garish Thomas-the-Tank-Engine lampshade (yes, yes, it was switched off; I am as neurotic about fire as the next woman), but it fell off.

- Overtired babies settle as badly as very energetic ones. If you keep a baby awake all day 'to get a good evening', you may end up with a hysterical, exhausted clinger at 6.30.

- Anyway, there is no need for a baby to be totally ready for instant sleep at bedtime. Some get into a cheerful habit of cooing and chuntering and chatting for up to an hour, unwinding after the day, happy in their cots.

- Cots and bedrooms have to be a treat, not a Colditz or a place of lonely exile. They should be special yet familiar. If babies never get the habit of bringing certain dear cuddlies and soft toys downstairs, these pleasant things become the inhabitants of a warm, drowsy, friendly world of blankets and lambskins and pictures on the wall. They are friends to greet again with joy at rest times and bedtimes. The trick is to stop the baby ever finding out that bed is actually a place where you thankfully dump him at the end of a long day, in the pious hope that he won't learn to escape from it. If you are mad enough to follow the advice of the doctor who wrote that temper-tantrums are best punished by 'shutting in his room', you could find that the panicky, angry vibrations build up and attach to the bedroom, and stay there for years.

- A useful tool in the process of making bed alluring is the baby alarm. Some parents loathe the idea of hearing every snort and sigh, and robustly claim that you can hear them anyway if they actually cry; but a good alarm (that is, one powerful enough not to distort sound but to pick up every rustle and sigh) is a brilliant device. It enables you to hear the first faint whimper, and whip in there quickly to stuff back whatever erring rag or teddybear has caused the sleepy dismay. It means that you can assess the mood of your child as he drifts off and wakes up (some babies witter happily for ages in bed night and morning – without the alarm we might think that 'Moo' and 'Quack' and 'Daddy said sod it bluggy car, sod it sod it' were cries of distress, not happy reminiscences of the day past). It means that you know if the child is sick, choking or croupy in the night. Paradoxically, for such a noisy instrument, a baby alarm can make you sleep better.

- Try not to bring a baby downstairs after bedtime once bedtime is established (around six months, if you're lucky). It is actually possible to con a toddler into thinking that you go to bed when he does. If he ever discovers the exciting adult world of evening, it could prove seductive enough to encourage cot-climbing and invasion. We kept this con-trick going for ages, and had quite a lot of evenings full of spacious, silent, infant-free liberty: a glittering prize. The occasional foray upstairs to sort out imbroglios with lost teddies, drinks-a-water, feet stuck in cot-bars etc. is a small price to pay.

- Penelope Leach has a golden, excellent piece of advice: to be always available 'but very boring' after bedtime. At every wail, up you go, and stand there boringly handing over the drink of water and being as dull *as* hell. Assuming there is no real reason for the baby to cry, except wanting your company, he will eventually find crying not worth the effort just in order to get this tedious zombie coming in and saying: 'Not asleep yet? Dear me, here's your nice teddy, night-night, then.' By 3 a.m. one can get very dull indeed.
- A cup of warm milk, taking over from the night breastfeed in the 20 minutes before bed, works both as a ritual and a sedative.
- Talking of rituals, elaborate ones will quite likely build up over the next few years without your encouraging them now; kissing every stuffed animal night-night in the right order and reciting the same three nursery rhymes while straightening the quilt exactly to the bed-corners will begin to pall on you when the child is pushing five. But one or two phrases can indicate even to a ten-month-old that bed is inevitable. 'Well … BEDFORDSHIRE,' says Daddy, in a particular tone of bonhomous desperation, and baby knows that this is it. The end of the day. Kismet. No chance of reprieve.

But, as I said before, all this will only irritate you if you are still in the middle of a terrible nightly battle. It may help to remember that what you are actually trying to do is to get the baby to stay in the cot without crying; not necessarily to go straight off to sleep. Accept that, and you're half-way; so a dim soft light, safe squashy toys, even a board book or two are quite acceptable inducements to offer. And there is the added advantage that if a baby likes playing in the cot in the evening, or looking at mobiles and pictures, he is more likely to do it in the morning, too. Then you, lying half-awake, will hear a broadcast of shrieks and giggles down the baby alarm. There are worse ways to wake up.

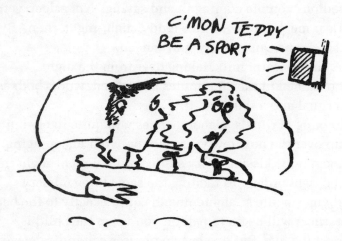

Chapter Five

The Leaving
of Little Ones

To this day, I can never step into the building which housed London Weekend Television without a wave of terror and panic sweeping over me. This has nothing to do with appearing on TV (which, compared to motherhood, is in fact a very restful experience); but it has everything to do with babies.

What happened was that one night, when my first child was about three months old, I was booked to record two editions of the panel game *Tell the Truth*. Since he had been happily taking the odd bottle of expressed milk, I decided for the first time to leave him behind, rather than make my usual straggling arrangements with carrycot, changing-bag, agency childminder meeting me in the dressing-room, and the rest of it. The engagement was from 5 p.m. until at least 10 p.m.; the studio audience, fellow-panellists and assorted competitors were all lined up. No substitutions were possible: *Tell the Truth* was, in a complicated medium, one of the most complicated recordings to arrange. I was a cog in that machine; I could not have pulled out, unless my child was mortally ill.

So what happened? At six o'clock (four hours to go, locked half an hour's drive from home in the great LWT fortress), I rang home.

Paul said: 'He's crying. He's just been screaming for half an hour. I can't do anything to stop him. He won't drink his milk. I don't know what to do.'

I have never panicked so comprehensively in my life. In seconds, I was awash with sweat and leaking milk, impervious to cool reason, aching precisely as if I had just delivered the baby over again; I was adrift and drowning in a stormy sea of tossing hormones. One of my fellow-panellists, an actress, to whom I am eternally grateful, hauled me away to sit down; we repaired my make-up, and got into the studio. Oddly, once the lights came on I managed the programme reasonably well; but every time there was a brief recording-break more sweat, milk and terror overcame me. Finally at ten o'clock I raced for a taxi, urged it desperately homeward, and ran into the house in tears to rescue my poor threatened baby.

Who had, of course, been peacefully asleep ever since ten past six.

Most mothers could tell you a story like that. Leaving a baby is painful, the first time; painful when it is to be for long; painful, at any age, when the baby is ill or upset or the minder is not your first choice. I have sat in tears on a train to London because I had left the children with a newly sacked nanny who – serving out her notice – had caused a bad-tempered row just as I left. How can you leave your tiny children with someone who hates you? I have dithered desperately between a toddler with a feverish cold and presenting a live radio programme 90 miles away. (How bad is the cold? Is it dangerous? Could it suddenly get worse? Will anybody ever employ me again if I rat out on a major programme just for a sniffly cold?) I have run out of petrol on a lonely country road, on my way home to breastfeed. I have dragged my husband away from a pompous formal Yacht Club dinner *(before the speeches,* gasp, shock, horror) because of an unformed and completely unjustified sense of foreboding about the baby back at home. I think, as a matter of interest, that this was the first time that the father in question fully realized that parenthood had changed everything, forever. Still, I was not lost to all sense of decency; I did wait until after the Loyal Toast to throw my wobbler. Oh, it is a dreadful business, leaving babies.

Dreadful, that is, when it isn't glorious! I have also known that inimitable lightness of step, running down the road with no buggy, no sling, no bag of baby wipes; getting to a wonderful office full of grown-ups whose noses don't run all the time. I have given little whoops of joy at going out to dinner without a carrycot, and skipped merrily around shops with both hands (and a whole mind) free after months of servitude. I have looked across railway carriages at a mob of whining infants, and praised heaven that not one single one of them is mine. And I have come back, refreshed, even after an hour or so, to take up the threads again.

If you can learn, and arrange, to leave babies behind sometimes, it adds a whole new zest to life. And if you *can't* learn to be away from them, both you and they are in for a nasty time if, for instance, you have a second one and go into hospital for it.

Even the most dedicated full-time home-based mother needs to learn the skills of handing over. So I have deliberately separated the subject from the thornier area of 'Working Motherhood'; and put it here, between babies and toddlers. For the earlier you start, the easier it is for all.

When I asked my panel of mothers, all perfectly sensible, loving, responsible women – some working, some not – about the best way to leave a baby to settle with a minder, nanny or relation for the morning, I got no sort of consensus.

'A firm cheerful goodbye,' said one. 'No shrieks, sobs or sad faces. Just go.'

Another briskly said, 'Don't waste time. Just go away and leave them.'

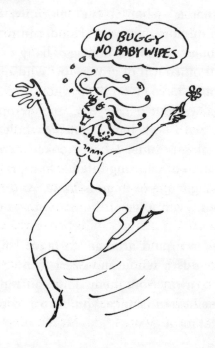

But another: 'Spend a lot of time settling in. Don't plonk the baby down straight away and leave.'

There was a strong lobby for food as a comforter: 'Leave her just starting a favourite biscuit,' was one piece of advice; another just wrote: 'Plug with food, dump and run!'

'Always say goodbye,' said one mother; while another, as firmly, advocated 'melting silently away while she's looking at something else'.

If you listened to all of them, you would get so confused that you'd burst into tears, upset your baby horribly, and lose all ways. However, *all of them are right.* This great truth struck me one day as I was sitting on the floor with my two-year-old, carefully explaining about Mummy's trip to London and how it would result in a toy helicopter tomorrow when he woke up from his afternoon nap; while at the same time frantically motioning to the nanny to distract the one-year-old while I sloped out to the car. Different ages, different babies, need entirely different leaving techniques. A little baby might be quite taken in by a dodge practised by several mothers – giving the minder your jumper to wear, or dousing her with your perfume ('Expensive, but worth it!'). But an *older* baby could be driven into screaming terror at such a substitution – my son got upset at the sight of another man with curly dark hair like his father's, when Daddy was away. New babies work on instinct; older ones reason that they only have one Mummy, who always comes back, but that substitutes are acceptable. A dressed-up substitute could actually be terrifying: Mummy, yet not Mummy. Aaagh!

Or take the business of 'melting away' while the baby looks elsewhere. This works fine, for months and months;

the actual moment of door-closing is so horrid that it makes sense to spare the baby that. But once a baby is beginning to reason things out, a moment comes (probably around 18 months) when if you keep 'melting' without a formal goodbye, he begins to suspect that you might 'melt' at any time without warning – and can't ever enjoy your company because he's wondering how long it will last.

Or take the 'one last game' technique: that depends on the child's precise mood as well as stage of development. Sometimes, making Mummy stay for one last story-on-a-knee is a pleasant confirmation of his great power over Mummy. Sometimes it prolongs the agony, and you should just leave.

So paradoxically, the better you know your baby and the closer you are, the easier it is to leave – because you know, precisely, to the closest nuance, how to manage it gracefully with least pain all round. The odds are that if you are careful about it, the pain will be minimal or non-existent. One of the most sensible pieces of advice I got, when I began, was: 'Don't expect the baby to mind you going, and don't be insulted if he doesn't.' Frankly, under 18 months old, a surprising number of babies are perfectly happy to spend a morning, even a day, with a reasonably familiar minder. I sometimes suspect they find it a nice change …

But your baby is your baby, and only you (and then, only if you are concentrating) can work out the best ways to leave him. Here are a few useful reflections for the moment of truth:

- Some recent research confirmed what most experienced parents probably knew: that even very young babies are capable of understanding that their parents love them very much. If you show enormous affection whenever you *do* see the child, he will actually find it easier to carry on in your absence. If you are allowing yourself to feel guilty, therefore miserable and artificially detached, the baby will know that, too, and won't like it.

- Even babies and toddlers who are left screaming with rage at their mother's departure generally settle down straight away when she goes. Which is more than can be said for the poor, stomach-churned mother weeping on her way to the bus stop. Some people have a system whereby the minder, as soon as the crying stops, puts a balloon or a flag at the window. Then Mum, out there in the rain, can look up with haggard face, like some heroine of a film about the French Resistance, see the all-clear, and go down the street rejoicing in *La Liberation.*

- Minders, nannies, grannies, neighbours etc. may not much enjoy being fully debriefed about exactly what happened when you went, what cheered the child up, what they did all day and whether the baby asked for Mummy; but you have got a perfect right to do it, every single time if you want to: you are building up a personal dossier on your child with, and without, your company.

- Really difficult babies sometimes settle down much better in their own home. A friend, only able to afford a communal childminder, actually persuaded one to come to her big rambling house, and bring her three other charges with her. They kicked the house around a bit, but the home-based baby enjoyed it, the childminder was quite glad of mornings away, and the

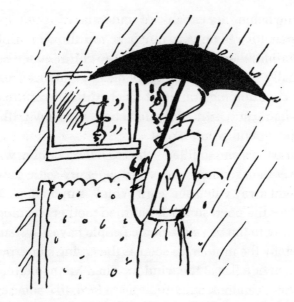

other parents didn't seem to mind. That was a rare arrangement, though.

- A good compromise between staying and melting away was the one I worked out when first handing over to a daily nanny at nine o'clock (baby three to nine months old). I would see her in, put the baby on her knee, and *wait for the first smile* of recognition. Smile over, I felt free to flit. The longest it ever took was twelve minutes, and I missed my train; but it made *me* feel better, anyway.
- There is nothing silly about briefing every babysitter and dayminder about every single emergency. You do feel a bit of a fool at times, though: one night I went out with the words: 'We're at the Horse Show, but in an emergency the local police would get us paged in the arena. The police and fire numbers are in the black book

by the telephone; so is the doctor's surgery and all the partners' home numbers. Ann down the road used to be a missionary nurse, and her husband has a good set of tools.' (This related to the time we thought he would have to use his tin-snips to get a cake-ring off Nicholas's head.) 'Nancy next door knows all about the trip-switch in the attic if there's a power cut; if Rose cries, it's probably because she's lost her muslin cuddly; if Nicholas needs any more Calpol he can't have it before 10.30. Oh, and if the house burns down, once you've got the children out please tell the firemen there's an orphan duckling in the cardboard box in the upstairs study, and could they get it out if possible, there's a ladder in the ...' .etc. You do feel a bit like James Thurber's auntie, who piled all her possessions outside the bedroom door every night so that burglars wouldn't break in and murder her, but a good handover briefing does somehow make for a more serene evening out.

- Another great comforter for absent parents is to have instilled into any minder the vital principle that in a medical emergency they ring the doctor first, before messing around trying to get through to you in some distant office with a jammed switchboard. And tell her not to be diffident: doctors are *paid* to be disturbed about the symptoms of small children. Once upon a time, I rushed a baby to hospital at 7.30 in the morning with a head wound. The doctor's surgery was shut; I had no transport, so I ran round the corner and made the police lend me a car and driver to the hospital. First the police kept saying, 'Oh, you want the ambulance service,' and I had to stamp my foot at

them; then, at the hospital, Casualty (full of morose
drunks) said, 'Oh, we haven't a doctor on until 8.30.' I
had to stamp that foot again, threaten to report them to
the GMC (is it the GMC? I wouldn't know, but nor did
the receptionist) and insist that – this being a hospital –
there damn well *must* be a doctor in it, somewhere, to
look at a two-month-old baby with blood coming out of
his head. I threatened to go walkabout, baby in arms,
and flag down the first white coat I saw. In five minutes
I got a doctor, and she stitched him up. Even the
morose drunks applauded, and the doctor herself said
she was glad I had put my foot down. But if I had been
a shy, polite, unassertive little 19-year-old *au pair*, I
might have sat there for an hour dabbing blood off the
baby's brow and wondering about concussion. Ever
afterwards, I chose babysitters and nannies with a
tough, mean, opinionated streak in their characters;
and reinforced it with precept and example. Someone
has to be 100 per cent on your baby's side.

- Overnight absences need a slightly different technique.
  Creeping off after babies are in bed can give you many
  hours' start – but watch like a hawk for any signs that
  they are starting to assume that you'll *always* go away if
  they dare to sleep – if so, stop doing it, quickly, or
  you've got a sleeping problem. Go away visibly, instead.
- Don't be horribly offended if the baby is nasty to you,
  or ignores you, after a longish absence. It is common,
  and passes. Absolutely dreadful while it lasts, though; I
  have hammered home from London, longing for my
  little ones, only to be met with a stony silence and an
  ostentatious draping of little arms round Nanny's or

Daddy's neck. There was generally a raging tantrum later, at bathtime, then we were all mates again.

- If you want to go away on holiday without the baby (working mothers rarely seem to do this; homebound mothers possibly need it more) it might pay to do so before 18 months old. As the two-year-old stage approaches, the child will mind more and more, have more of a sense of time passing, and draw more erroneous conclusions about being deserted forever. A nice fortnight abroad while your one-year-old or younger baby stays home with Granny could be a tonic. But a nice fortnight abroad followed by six weeks of night-waking, tantrums and heartbreaking queries of 'Does Mummy love 'oo?' is more like a draught of hemlock.
- Finally, let me quote my mother, left overnight for the first time in charge of both babies. With a seraphic smile, she said, 'We will *survive,* dear. I can promise nothing about putting these modern vests on them the right way up, or working that microwave thing of yours, but we will all still be here in the morning, perfectly happy in our own way.' And they were.

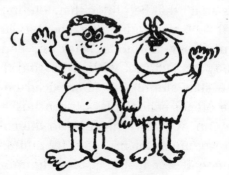

• •

Chapter Six

Double Shift:
Working Mothers

Despite repeated government attempts to get British mothers of small children back to work, and an enormous change in expectations over the past 20 years or so, nobody you ever meet seems to think very highly of mothers who head back to full-time work while their children are very small. With good reason, it is a major source of guilt: even a part-time working mother can be reduced to tears by some earth-mother offering a pitying smile, with 'Oh, it must be awful for you,' and 'Of course, everyone's priorities are *so* different, but they're only little for such a short time, after all, *such* important years ...'

Employers aren't that helpful, either, tending to suspect that you will feel pretty different about *their* priorities once your motherly hormones kick in, and childless colleagues may suspect (not without reason) that you are now going to start sloping off home dead on time, and needing time off for school plays. Even husbands sometimes display unsupportive hostility to the co-breadwinner ('Doesn't say much for *me*, does it,' mutter their own ancient hunter-gatherer instincts, '*her* dumping the kids and going off to work'). Even apparent allies can speak with forked tongues: articles on working motherhood concentrate markedly on school runs, latch-keys, nativity plays, gym kit and other paraphernalia belonging entirely to over-fives; and every time someone says, 'I think you're *marvellous,* doing it all,' you can hear, faint but distinct, the unspoken addition: '… you supercilious, selfish cow.'

If you entrust your child to a minder, righteous mothers sniff and imagine some squalid baby-farmer. If you have a nanny, people infuriatingly assume that you never touch your baby, night or day, and are stinking rich to boot. If you break right out and take the baby along to your place of work with you, feeding it surreptitiously in your lunch-hour, even more hostility builds. You might as well accept that a mother's place is in the wrong. Never more so than if she works.

Why do it, then? Why not give those few years entirely to motherhood, and go back later? There are many possible reasons. I must admit that my original motive – largely financial, for we are both freelancers – was reinforced by a conviction that I couldn't go from day to day, isolated with tiny children, and stay sane. After a while, I was less sure of that as I would sit at my keyboard, worrying about some particularly hairy dash across London from train to studio (a dash, so that I could linger at home to get the babies up and kiss them goodbye), and see out of my window a care-free girl in jeans, romping around on a sunlit lawn with my two children, earning the money which I would earn by struggling through the rush-hour. Later, the nanny would be out for a cup of coffee and more romping at the mother-and-toddler group, and I would be miles away,

having a long and tedious argument with a stubborn magazine editor. The grass often looked a lot greener on the
other side. Still, I daresay, there were people down at the
toddler group, wiping tears and snot off their discontented
offspring, who thought my life glamorous and desirable.
Indeed, there were also mornings when driving away from
the whole teething, captious, unappreciative circus was
pure delight. But you must decide: and try, if you can, not
to make the decision irreversible. There are families, and
times, when mothers and very small children are simply
better off staying together, on less money.

Money might be the important bit, though. In Britain
nearly half of mothers with children under two do some
kind of work, and they are not all doing it for personal
fulfilment – not by a long chalk. Some do it, rather desperately, to 'stay on the career ladder' in case they can't get
work again later. Many do it quite simply to put food on
the family table and pay the mortgage, or rent, and taxes.
You need not be on the breadline to need work – perhaps
just living in a house whose mortgage keeps getting higher
as interest rates rise, or married to a man whose wage is in
jeopardy, or to a father who longs for the freedom to soft-
pedal his own career and have time with the children
instead. You may be working to save for a burning family
ambition – to get out of the city, perhaps, to emigrate, to
buy a boat, to build a granny-flat.

Whatever the reason, there is absolutely no advantage
in being guilty about it. If you're really guilty, and feel that
it is doing damage to your particular relationship with
your particular child – then do something drastic. Sell the
big house, take in ironing or typing, work at night and

mother all day, become a paid childminder yourself, take a lodger – anything. If the thought of these options is even more appalling and damaging than your present life, the odds are that you are already doing the best thing possible; so why be guilty?

If you work entirely for your own pleasure (a few do) all you can do is to make sure that you spend every penny you can on providing a long-term, loving, brilliant substitute for yourself while you do it. Every day, somewhere, a natural mother beats up her children or neglects them; while somewhere else, a foster-mother or a nanny makes a small child entirely happy. There is not necessarily anything magical about natural motherhood. Only the overall responsibility is inalienable. And if you try to deny that responsibility – the duty at least to *arrange* 24-hour love and attention – you will probably make yourself miserable anyway. If you don't care, then you are too wicked for the scope of this book …

But, as a railway guard once said to me when I offered to get out and push the train into the next station, 'It don't gener'ly come to that.' To combine earning and early mothering merely involves a gigantic, years-long compromise, and the almost total destruction of your free time. It takes a lot of managing, and a lot of sacrifice. It is not a selfish option, except very rarely indeed. But nobody is going to feel very sorry for you. While few will be rude enough to use the words 'money-grabbing' to your face, many will mutter them from the security of their sink. They will forget that you, too, have a sink; and that it is always waiting for you at the end of the long day.

The working options divide up pretty neatly:

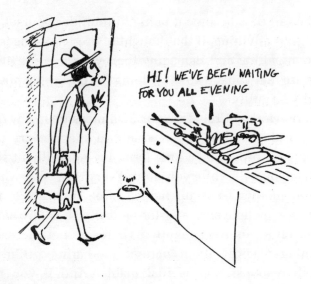

1. Working away from home

Off to the office she goes! Designer Woman, briefcase in hand, dashes off importantly in the Volvo, kissing a row of rosy little smiling faces, briefing the rosy, smiling nanny on which homemade delicacies to take out of the well-ordered freezer for the children's lunch. She trips off to work, where her secretary waits for the first batch of razor-sharp decisions on the morning's post. What a Superwoman! Don't we all admire her every pinstripe, as she grins confidently out of the advertisements and Working-woman Lifestyle Profiles at us!

Well, no, actually, we don't. We hate her guts. We coo and burble to our babies until ten minutes before the train, pull on the least unclean clothes from the bedroom floor, stuff our feet into scraped and heel-less shoes, and tell the white-faced nanny that if her toothache gets worse, she is to leave the baby next door with instructions to pass him on to number 13 at four o'clock when next door has to get her own child from school, because she's only got one baby-seat in the car, and that if the dentist says she has to have the tooth out tomorrow, Nanny must ring *immediately* before 12.30 so that Mummy can cancel the Goldsmith-Securities Conference and be able to stay home half the morning because next door *would* have obliged, only she's got an incontinent auntie coming to stay and can't do mornings …

Then we run for the train, and strap-hang, heart pounding, wondering whether the cat got fed, whether Nanny will faint with pain at her wisdom tooth while the baby crawls into the fireplace; we arrive hopeless and exhausted, fit only for coffee and a grumble, and find all hell broken loose because we decided to leave a meeting dead on 5.30 yesterday in order to be home for bathtime. We do all this, and curse Mrs Imaginary Superwoman's imaginary calm.

Genuinely bombproof childcare arrangements do not exist. The rich do better: but even if you had a nanny *and* a housekeeper, the day would come when one had measles and the baby screamed in terror of the other. Even if you have the world's best neighbours, the day will come when they have all gone off together to the Townswomen's Guild Jam Tea, just as the *au pair* runs off with the coalman and Daddy goes on business to Peru. So the day will come when there is no option but to take a carrycot, or a toddler and a packet of crayons (pray God not a potty too), into the office for an hour or so. I have yet to work *anywhere* where it hasn't happened once (although generally the mothers who do it most freely are those highest in the pecking order. Madam Boss's baby is one thing; Miss

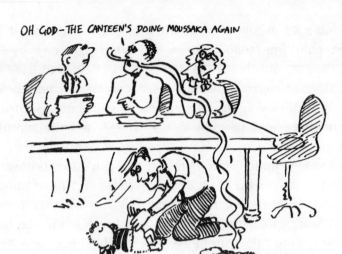

OH GOD-THE CANTEEN'S DOING MOUSSAKA AGAIN

Supersecretary's baby is quite another). But if the human race is to continue, and babies are to be looked after kindly, and women with talents are to use them – then someone, somewhere, is going to be inconvenienced by the odd gurgling carrycot behind the filing cabinets. The head of a Radio 4 department once changed his son's nappy on the floor in the course of a large meeting. He says that nobody noticed, which was pretty impressive, considering that the meeting was actually in his own office and he was chairing it. My own childcare arrangements once collapsed dramatically and left me obliged to feed Nicholas during a meeting with two senior police officers, the Controller of Radio 4, and others. The feeding was most discreet. Not so the subsequent loud hiccupping. But we all survived.

On the whole, though, it is still better not to bring even an atmosphere of baby-talk into most offices, on most days. The odd lapse is one thing; a constant aroma of sicked-up milk and emotional strain is another. Some useful rules of thumb for maintaining your credibility are:

- Learn to change pace. You rapidly discover that when you dash back into the house in the evening, you are required to slow down to a lackadaisical baby pace, overemphasizing words, repeating silly jokes and noises, patiently removing the same little hand again and again from the same light fitting. What is absolutely vital is to remember, in the morning, to *reverse the procedure* and speed up again. I never laugh, any more, at the old tale of the woman who sat next to a fascinating man at an official dinner, and noticed too late that she had cut up all his meat for him. Not since I was guest speaker at a Royal Naval Volunteer Reserve dinner and the port was circulating on a silver gun-carriage, and I pushed it away from me into the centre of the table lest an imaginary baby should knock it over.
- Don't keep ringing home. Give home *your* number, instead. Train your babysitter never to say, 'It's the nanny,' if this produces unkind groans in your office. Try: 'It's personal – I'm returning her call,' or something neutral like that. Having said this, I must confess to having inflicted the following one-sided conversation on the very chic, very baby-free main office of the *Tatler* one day:

'Claire? Is anything wrong? He's WHAT? He's not! *A tooth!* It can't be! I never saw – no, really! That's amazing, that's wonderful, give him a kiss from me!'

Confirmed bachelors shuddered delicately in the background, and willowy fashion-writers shrugged. Only a sub-editor, her own children long grown up, flashed me a wily and conspiratorial smile …

- 'Never mention children at work, unless asked,' said an executive mother. 'And then be extremely brief. Men never talk about their children at work.' Well, in some offices that is true enough; but I have worked in a local radio station full of New Men, where the women were mustard-keen and career-minded, and the men rambled on and on about placentas and potties.

- 'Wear nail polish,' said one mother of three. 'Gives an impression of efficiency and time to spare. So does make-up.' Sexist, alas, but true.

- If you use a childminder, pack up your baby-kit in bulk every weekend, so you don't spend every morning fretting about spout-mugs and disposable nappies.

- And if you *have* had to leave a crisis at home, 'Put on your make-up, telephone frequently but covertly, and if you can't cope – develop a psychosomatic headache and leave.'

2. Working part-time

This is a good option for mothers (and for fathers, too; one day the family with two half-jobs may be commonplace). Already there is more acceptance of job-sharing, or flexi-time, or shiftwork, or anything irregular that gives you an income and an escape valve, without blocking you off permanently from daytime weekday life at home. The snag is that unless you have a good ration of help, the 'part' of time that you work inevitably turns out to be *your* part – the bit that used to be free, or free-ish. Plenty of women dash home from night shifts to look after babies all day; a few fathers do it too. It is not fun. If you can afford any help at all, even a trusty schoolgirl to wheel a pram round for an hour a day, it helps. Job-sharing is getting more voguish in Britain; employers have realized that they actually get one and a half employees for the price of one, since each tries hard to outshine the other.

A very new animal indeed is emerging to match: the job-share-share-a-nanny, who flits between households as mothers go in to work and out again. This is a flimsy but economical structure, if you can build it and can both get on with the communal nanny. Like one of those spindly contraptions which used to cross the Channel in air-races, the arrangement feels as if it could never fly, but it some-times does.

3. Working at home

On the face of it, a wonderful compromise. There you are, like William Wordsworth, sitting at your worktable surrounded by your children playing happily. You earn money and respect, without moving away from the hearth. You dictate your own schedule. You need never miss bathtime or leave a feverish child. You can get up and walk ten feet and hug the baby and walk back and be at work again. Magic.

Some heroic women manage to work at home – sewing, typing, proofreading, writing, computer programming, doing crafts, even running a small business – without any help at all with their preschool children. 'I get into the playpen,' said one, 'and work there.' But if there is a sudden quiet from the direction you last saw the baby, you will quite rightly leap from the playpen, heart hammering, and find the brat eating Vim or dismembering a first edition.

'Story and song cassettes help for half an hour or so,' said another homeworker.

'No, hopeless,' said another. 'Only ten minutes' peace, then it's "Want my very own typewriter", and whining for a walk.'

The general chorus said: 'The AFTERNOON SLEEP is the thing.' It can extend, as all cunning, manipulative mothers know, far beyond the need for actual sleep; I remember being put in my room for a 'rest' until school-age, and I'm not sure that it didn't continue in the holidays, until we were about eight. I was grown up before I realized exactly who was having the 'rest' during all those hours.

Still, it is pleasant enough at any age to spend an hour in a dim room with a book and a musical-box. The only thing about afternoon rests, though, is that if you drop them more than two days running, you may have a battle on your hands to reinstate them. And a nasty side-effect of trying to work, and be sole mother, at home is that you can start really to resent your poor babies waking up; resent their cheery coos and shouts for Mummy; and positively dislike their climbing on your knee uninvited. This is not a good way to be a happy mother. You actually start to envy the office-worker who, at home, can be 100 per cent thrilled and enthusiastic about her children.

No; you can work more effectively, and be a nicer mother, if you have some sort of babysitter or nanny while you work. If you are genuinely at home *all* the time, you can get by with a younger, cheaper version – a 'learner nanny', perhaps, or a bright 16-year-old; but you need someone.

(Preferably someone who switches effortlessly into ironing-and-dusting mode, like a multi-purpose computer, during the afternoon sleep. There are few things more infuriating than a nanny lying supine on her bed watching daytime TV for the duration of a two-hour infant nap.)

If you can't justify a whole nanny, you could have a string of babysitters, to take children out for healthy walks at set times; or join in the fearful 'swopping' system which operates in middle-class neighbourhoods. This is a sort of nightmare chain-letter, in which you send off your own children for three mornings a week and then suddenly, on Friday, you win the jackpot of twelve small children for lunch, and no quarter asked or given. One old friend of mine used to be particularly bitter about this, because she discovered that everyone else in the lunch-giving chain delegated the whole lot to their *au pair*, leaving her the only genuine Mummy in the system. She felt she ought to have got a bonus for experience, decent food and a comprehensible accent.

Even with a full-time nanny in the house, though, there are hazards about trying to work at home:

- It is nine o'clock. Nanny clocks on; you prepare to do the same in your study; your toddler thinks differently. He has got a cold, and wants Mummy. Unwilling to make an issue of it, you let him sit at your feet. By the time he is calm enough to be transferred, Nanny has mysteriously vanished with the other child on an extended walk.
- The telephone rings. You have splashed out on an extension in your working-room, but Nanny is not quick enough and your child gets to it first, and begins rambling on about Great Big 'Normous Tipper-Trucks,

or poo-poos, to your boss. The incident I most wish to forget was when Edward Heath, former Prime Minister, happened to ring back personally to give me a brief quote for an article. The two-year-old entertained the poor man for several minutes with a tuneless serenade on the Toot-A-Floot and a string of unconnected remarks about ducks. Oh, the shame.

- You are doing well, nearly finished a tricky piece of work. Nanny knocks on the door. The kitchen drain is blocked and overflowing into the baby's sandpit. Nobody at Norland gave instructions about unblocking drains, and 'heavy domestic work' was excluded from her contract. Since absolutely nothing is excluded from *your* lifelong contract, you get in there with the plunger while Nanny gathers the little ones to her skirts with many a hygienic sniff and mutter. It was never like this at Lady X's.

- There is a bang and a scream. You sit huddled over your work, wondering what to do. There is an awful silence. You go out to the kitchen, to find all serene. You make a cup of tea, still wondering what the bang and scream were, but are unwilling to give the

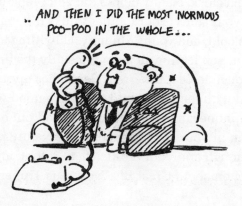

.. AND THEN I DID THE MOST 'NORMOUS POO-POO IN THE WHOLE...

impression that you don't trust your *au pair*. You notice it is nearly lunchtime. Thirty minutes lost.

- It is lunchtime. You have no firm arrangement with your nanny about whether it is her job to feed you, as well as the baby. In fact, you want a cheese sandwich at the desk. But on emerging to make it, you find that she has made a beautiful lasagne, and you are included. She is also sitting in a marked sulk because you are Late and the food has got Cold. You choke it down, try to pacify her by doing all the washing-up, and take your child upstairs for his nap. Two hours lost, and you return to the typewriter with a looming dread of Nanny resigning in dudgeon just when you have a vital deadline to meet. Then the local playgroup organizer 'phones, 'because I knew you'd be home ...'
- You are deeply immersed in work. The 'phone rings. It is a friend with a child the same age, asking yours round to paddle in his pool. Socially blackmailed, you realize uneasily that it is you, not Nanny, who is wanted to gossip at the poolside. You go, and lose half a day's work. Conversely:
- The local nanny-mafia, plus charges, are meeting in your house for tea. You creep out to join in, anxious to find out what company your child is keeping (office mothers never get a chance to see, so miss nothing).
- It is the end of the day. The children are in bed, Daddy is home, Nanny is off, peace returns. But since all the above disruptions have happened in the same week, you are way behind; instead of sitting down to supper, television and matrimonial grunts about the past day, you go sadly back into your study, and work until half

past one. Simply because the work is there. And it always will be.

But working at home need not be all that bad. Hidden in that doleful list of frustrations are the basic ground-rules for doing it happily: get a helper who understands your life and takes small crises in her stride; get an extension telephone which unplugs to foil tiny hands; set clear working hours and be curt with time-wasting domestic callers during those hours; allow yourself to knock off at another set hour, and turn the key on your workroom.

All this still leaves leeway for the sad, sniffly child who wants to sit under the desk for half an hour; why else are you making such an effort to earn your living at home? If all is well between a child and his paid minder, he won't join you often or for very long; a deeply boring Mummy is quite easily abandoned for a painting, playdough-slinging, paddling-pool-inflating, all-singing all-dancing babysitter.

Being a working mother has huge advantages; apart from the financial security, and the ability to make a few decisions in the outside world, it teaches you whole new disciplines. On a good day, you really do feel like Superwoman. It trains you in the art of dividing your work into that which can be done with a child under the desk, that which can be done while breastfeeding, and that which genuinely requires total freedom from anyone under 21. It teaches you incredible concentration: I used to string paperclips by the hour; now, the moment I have an all-clear on the domestic front, I fling myself savagely on the keyboard and get going. It can make you more loving and tolerant of your children – I used to get back from one office and jump on my son in glee, saying, 'Do you know, I haven't met anyone as nice as you *all day*.' (It is harder to say that at the weekends, after 12 hours' concentrated whingeing and sibling-bashing.) Working, if you can stand the pace, is exhilarating. But when you distil all the experience down, two important problems remain to be solved – even in the most ideal balance of work and home. Both are emotional.

The first concerns the child, or children. If you lose touch with the daily life of a small child – particularly before it can really talk and tell – that child is much harder to handle and to enjoy when you do see each other. Every weekend you can watch little fiends flinging themselves on the floor of teashops and supermarkets, playing up Mummy and Daddy in a way that would astonish Nanny if she could see it. It is a sign of love, and relief, and indignation at the paucity of Mummy except at weekends. It is hard to bear, when you have looked forward all week to being a mother again.

But you can cheat the syndrome, to some extent, by crafty planning of your time at home. If you keep on covering key times in the child's day, you stay in close touch on fewer hours than a full-time mother. For instance, we *always,* even if a nanny was living in, got the babies up in the morning, dressed them, and did breakfast. If I was going away, I sometimes even got them up earlier. At the other end of the day, you can take over for bathtime (always a good mothering time, with all that nakedness and laughter) and a sacrosanct half-hour or so before bed. I don't believe in the get-out phrase 'quality time' because a child may not want to bond with you to order, by the clock. But during their time with you, you can concentrate: not watching the news, but building Duplo castles or bouncing babies on a knee. The key moments at morning and evening weigh far heavier in the scales than treble the time elsewhere in the day.

Add to that all the odd moments you can – an appearance at lunchtime if you work at home, a trip in the car to do some photocopying, an occasional bus ride to your office and home again with Nanny – and you can build up a considerable bank of goodwill and confidence to offset the risk of those weekend furies. If you are, in addition, happy and jokey at breakfast rather than snappish and preoccupied with loading your handbag and putting on your camouflage makeup, the value doubles again.

The other problem is your own. The plain fact is that there is *no stretch at all* in the system; no 'give', except in you. Whatever time you carve out of your work belongs to the children, and vice versa. Fathers seem better able to carve themselves a niche of peace and privacy; mothers are lousy at it. I asked a selection of earning mothers, 'How do you get any time to yourself?' and the answers came various, and occasionally bitter:

'Don't know. Perhaps by walking out on the whole shooting-match?'

'Use the late nights. Completing this questionnaire of yours has meant three sessions during the small hours.'

'Tube-train journeys are surprisingly restful; lunch-hours can be blissfully private. Grab time when you have it.'

'The answer is entirely geographical – get away from work and child. A boat? Or tennis? Neither child nor typewriter can possibly appear on a club tennis court.'

'Join something which regularly takes you out of the house. A club, class, anything.'

'Once a fortnight I have a Turkish bath, shampoo, manicure and massage. It is blissful having someone else do all that for *you* for a change.' (I can well appreciate this one. Lying in the bath one night I came over quite faint at the realization that I was responsible for cutting 60 nails: 20 of mine on fingers and toes, 20 on each child ...)

'I feel too guilty to enjoy anything if I offload the children when I don't have to.'

'Anything, anything, so long as it is physically stretching. Keep-fit, tennis – or we've got an allotment!'

The last two sum up the problem, for me. Just as, when the babies were newborn, I could bear to let them grizzle while I served their interests – changed a cot or hung up washing – yet couldn't tolerate the same mild grizzling while I read a Sunday paper, so a year later I found it impossible to go off for a selfish private swim or walk. Going off to work is all right; going out on pleasure feels terrible. Yet the need for rough, physical, arm-swinging childfree exercise is overwhelming. A 'walk' with a buggy (shoulders rounded in defeat, little tripping steps), or with a dawdling two-year-old, is not a real walk at all. Most babycare is a matter of tittupping around in a limited space, making gentle movements and lifting heavy weights for short distances. This does not blow off any steam; it makes you tired in a snappish, irritable, unhealthy way. So does sitting in an office; the combination of both can drive you crazy. I was sent by *Punch* once to row 13 miles up the Thames like Jerome K. Jerome, and my two companions couldn't understand why I insisted on keeping an oar the whole way, instead of resting at the steering-lines: it was the sheer joy of physical exertion without tiny grabbing hands to ruin my swing, or fragile heads to watch out for.

So the occasional burst of private activity (or, if you prefer, private sloth) is worth planning for when you organize yourself back to work. This is a counsel of perfection; the balancing act between guilt at not hurrying home, and irritation at not having any private pleasures, is not one which I have ever quite mastered. One high-powered friend has a high-powered solution; she refuses to go on any company trip unless the hotel has a pool. 'It is', she says, 'the only guilt-free swimming I get, without a nervous little frog in armbands to slow me down.' Even then, I happen to know that the poor soft sap sometimes gazes tearfully out of rooftop restaurants in exotic places, thinking how much her three-year-old son would have enjoyed the lifts.

The trouble is, she's right: he would have. Knowing this, I actually took my 20-month-old son on a business trip to Plymouth once, complete with nanny, and we all shared a vast room in the Holiday Inn. What with the nanny lurching back in the small hours after a night out with half the Navy, and Nicholas getting overexcited about the bouncy bouncy beds, and Room Service forgetting to warm the milk for breakfast, it was all pretty intense.

The only thing none of us suffered from was guilt.

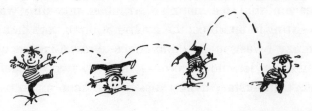

- -

Chapter Seven

A Tale of
Two Nannies

Once upon a time there was a nice young pregnant couple: let us call them Simon and Sarah. Once a week, when they had puffed and stretched their way through the natural-childbirth classes, they would go home to supper and discuss the management of their future family life. Sarah wanted to continue her career; Simon didn't want to be married to a housewife. In perfect agreement, they laid their plans: a nanny would be found at leisure, and employed for two weeks before the actual return to work. They knew exactly where other people went wrong when employing nannies, and joined in deploring their various friends who underpaid, were rude, exploited the girls and expected the husband's shirts to be ironed. (Simon had *always* done his own. He was a New Man.) Their nanny would suffer none of these indignities: she would be carefully chosen, reasonably well paid, trusted and consulted. There would be an easy atmosphere of give-and-take: if Sarah had a crisis at work, the girl would gaily stay on duty until late. If the nanny wanted a long weekend with her boyfriend, Sarah would understand. There would be frankness, and generosity, and loyalty.

As he dozed off, Simon would briefly entertain a separate little dream: of an old-fashioned, lightly starched, frumpy family retainer. In his dream, she brought his clean gurgling son to play with him, and waited smilingly behind the chair with a damp flannel to neutralize any infantile stickiness before it reached his jacket. Nanny would keep the kitchen surfaces clear and gleaming, pick up stray socks, and probably (this thought came *very* quietly, and sneakily, just before he fell asleep) she would *insist* on ironing his shirts ...

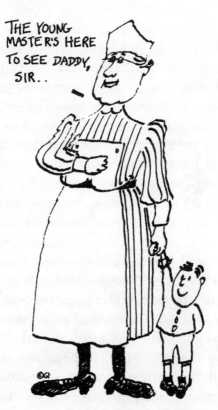

THE YOUNG
MASTER'S HERE
TO SEE DADDY,
SIR..

Sarah dreamed of a cross between a hospital nurse – omniscient about burps and teething – and a new best friend. She imagined a cheerful, competent girl, in jeans and sweatshirts, perhaps with a jolly Sloane Ranger background; or perhaps a motherly country girl, engaged to a policeman. Nanny would be welcome to bring her friends to the house – so that Sarah, hurrying home from work, would bump into well-spoken young men and girls, who would whisk politely upstairs to wait in Nanny's room before taking her out bowling, but who would admire the house and the child. A family community would be born – Simon and Sarah and baby and Nanny and these cheerful young droppers-in. Except that, of course, they wouldn't call her 'Nanny'! Christian names all round! Of course!

And both would fall asleep with their separate fantasies, until that inevitable night when Sarah shook Simon awake, picked up her neatly packed suitcase, rang the hospital and set off on the great adventure.

The advertisement in *The Lady* mentioned an 'airy family house' in a fashionable suburb, and specified a 'loving, responsible nanny' for 'Damien, 6 mths'. Simon had wanted to put 'nanny/mother's help', but Sarah was horrified. A mother's help, to her, was a sluttish, moronic foreigner without the brains to be a real nanny. It was an insult to her imaginary best friend. Besides, the two extra words would have meant dropping the bit about the 'busy executive mother' or paying another tenner. So 'nanny' it was; and 78 replies came in the first week.

They were a little shaken by the first round of telephone calls. They learned that every woman who can do nothing else thinks that – being a woman – she can look after children. After bruising encounters with an elderly Scottish alcoholic, a shifty-looking girl with two years unaccountably missing from her curriculum vitae, twenty hopeful sixteen-year-olds (Sarah had forgotten to specify any age) and a vacant-looking punk who, asked *how* she would entertain the baby, said, 'Oh, ride round 'n' round on the tube, mainly,' Sarah felt her nerve beginning to crack. Part of the trouble was that she felt she owed each applicant at least a half-hour interview, even if the first words on the 'phone convinced her they couldn't mind a budgerigar with any safety. Simon took over, censored the rest with brisk male ruthlessness, and gave her the last ten names to interview. They weren't quite what Sarah had envisaged; but all ten would have been perfectly accept-able. Especially after the punk and Mad Maggie frae Glasgow. Mindful of the experience of a friend who had interviewed rigorously and talked about Montessori water-play, development of prehensility and Transitional Comfort Objects, and who had nevertheless ended up with a girl who fled with all the household silver at the end of a fortnight, Sarah tried to relax and choose a girl who just seemed pleasant, honest and fond of babies. She found a sweet-eyed lass of 20, signed her on, and fell sobbing with relief into Simon's arms.

Gradually, life fell into its new pattern. They got used to the unnerving little scanties dripping over the bath, to finding the radio tuned to reggae stations they never knew existed, to communal breakfasts and all the small intru-sions which go with resident nannies. The baby thrived. Sarah found that if she actually mentioned a piece of tidy-ing-up, or washing, then it got done; if she didn't, it stayed undone. Often she was too tired and preoccupied to mention it; and, after all, the dear baby was happy; so she did it herself.

As young Damien grew older, and began to eat mushy food, Sarah would leave recipe books for babies around the place, and make bright conversation about the super-iority of homemade lunches; but could never quite bring herself to ask whether baby or nanny had eaten the contents of the baked-bean tins which she found in the kitchen bin most evenings. Trust, loyalty, a Good Relationship, she would think; and Damien seemed very contented. It was a pity that Sarah spent so much of the evening clearing up and cooking wholefood dishes for next day's lunch; she would have liked to join Simon as he played with Damien before bed; but everything was going so smoothly it seemed unwise to rock the boat. If Nanny took offence and walked out, Damien would be heartbroken, wouldn't he? And her job wouldn't stand a fortnight's absence for interviewing, not at the moment. So she toiled on. Nanny seemed very contented, after all ...

How long this would have continued nobody will ever know. But biology took a hand. Sarah, slightly to her surprise, found herself pregnant again. The sweet-eyed girl went a bit thoughtful; stayed a few months, then sweetly gave notice and left for Oman and the promise of vast riches, one princeling only to amuse, and a resident cook and housekeeper.

This time, unable to face the *Lady* process again, Simon insisted they use an agency. They also decided to specify a formal training, NNEB at the least, and to include some general domestic help. With a fine sense of being in

control, and a fervent resolution not to spend any more
evenings cleaning the highchair, Sarah interviewed the
three 'real' nannies pre-selected by the agency. Their references glowed; their hair was tidy; their fingernails immac-
ulate. Sarah chose one who spoke to Damien with a fine
professional coo in her voice, but firmly moved his hand
from the light switch with a kindly 'Little boys *never*
touch electricity.' As Damien generally touched everything he saw, all the time, this impressed Sarah hugely.
Nanny made only one request (pausing to tell Damien that
little boys *never* pull Mummy's hair): and that was that
she be formally called 'Nanny'. Simon gave a quiet, satis-
fied smile, and pulled thoughtfully at his loose cuff-
button.

The house ran like clockwork. Sarah would get back
from work to find a gleaming, clinical kitchen, the airing-
cupboard shelves freshly lined, curtains made and hanging where no curtains had hung before. Simon's knickers
were ironed to within an inch of their life, his shirts stiff.
Damien was whisked through three pairs of ironed dungarees a day, and operated to a strict timetable. The new
baby, once Sarah went back to work again, could be found
at the end of the day, looking a little baffled, in a frilled
white muslin bib, sucking a freshly sterilized rattle.

How the atmosphere began to curdle was a mystery at
first. Still dreaming of give-and-take, Sarah had not bothered
with a written contract; indeed Nanny did so many extra
little jobs at first that it would have been an embarrassment.

Why, she was often at the sink at 8 p.m. scrubbing
something that they had never even known needed scrubbing. So, of course, Sarah let her go off for appointments

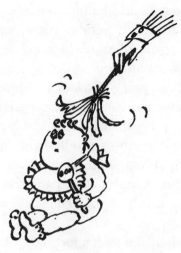

with her doctor, and her dentist, and her osteopath, and her hairdresser even, and took time off work herself to mind the babies. When the round of appointments ended, Nanny appeared one day to mention 'my half-day for this week'. Baffled, Sarah realized that the time off had somehow become a right rather than a concession; and that if a foot was not put down now, she would have a nanny on a four-and-a-half-day week.

The foot was never put down: Sarah decided that her mother could take the babies on Friday afternoons. Nanny, after all, did so much extra. Wasn't she working at nine o'clock last night, cleaning out the holes in the Duplo bricks in case the baby should suck them? Simon began to be quite rude about it, wishing to God the girl would go off duty, even ironing his own shirts as a gesture of protest. But Nanny was impervious. She was either there when you didn't want her, or off for a long weekend when you did. And Sarah was worried about poor Nanny, anyway:

she was often so exhausted after the week's work that she got a migraine attack on Sunday night, and couldn't get back from the weekend until Monday lunchtime. Poor Nanny, she did work so hard!

After nearly a year of Nanny, Simon and Sarah frequently screamed at each other, occasionally threatening divorce. They began to dislike the house and dread coming home. Damien began to be irritatingly clingy; the younger baby short-tempered. They never associated any of this with Nanny, only with parenthood; for Nanny continued to coo firmly at the babies and scrub worktops with Milton.

It was only when she took a fortnight's holiday that the penny dropped. Suddenly the house was free of a malevolent presence; Sarah muddled along, Simon burned his own collars and cuffs and learned to like his boxer-shorts crumpled; Damien and the baby seemed quite unperturbed by her absence, and their parents began to see the funny side of life again. After a week of exhausting, giggling, chaotic parenthood, they even got up the courage to sack Nanny and begin again.

You can write your own ending to the story. Perhaps Sarah realized that she was such a congenital doormat that she would be happier at home not employing anybody at all; perhaps they tried again and found a treasure – a friendly, willing, sensible girl who didn't have a taste for playing psychological games, and stayed for years. Perhaps things got worse, and they were taken in by one of the real hardcases who float around on the nanny market – the girls Jane Reed, of the Nanny Service, described to me:

'One was a thief. I knew about her, but another agency sent her out to a job; when she walked out, the mother rang me and said, "My nanny's just gone!" I said, "Oh dear, what was her name?" And when she told me, I said, "Go straight to your handbag – check your credit cards." And she did, and they were gone. And the girl was picked up later, but she'd already got into another job and cleaned out the jewellery … Then there was another girl, black-listed now, but she still carries references – she left a baby in a cot with a bottle, and it got fluid in its lungs and stopped breathing; and a month later when it came out of hospital the same thing happened again – but the mother was blackmailed into writing a reference. And then there was …'

No, no, stop, stop. We can all imagine the horror nannies, and the only way to ward them off is to take immense care in checking references (*speak* to previous employers, assess what they're really saying behind the stock phrases) and to watch any new minder carefully – either in person, or by briefing homebound neighbours, Granny etc. to keep popping in during the first months.

What is harder to anticipate is the psychological problem of employing a stranger in your own home, to look after your precious children. For a start, she will probably be much younger than you, and of a different background and character (well, she wants to spend all day with babies and you clearly don't). Add to that the fact that you, child of a servantless generation, have probably never employed a domestic before; and the fact that any third person, sharing a house with a young couple, is going to need a social and probably a sex life of her own. That

demure lass talking so enthusiastically about child development at the interview may well have a huge, aggressive,
biker boyfriend; or worse, several rival huge aggressive
biker boyfriends. That respectable, 35ish career-nanny
may be a career-nanny only because she is having a
prolonged affair with a married man from Cheadle, and
his wife may turn up one day on your doorstep.

Actually, I think I do not much mind queues of brawl-
ing bikers (or, in our case, a gormless GI from the local
USAF base paying calls at 8.30 on a Saturday morning
while the nanny hid in her room telling us to put him off).
I would even put up with the occasional enraged wife. At
least these diversions only affect the nanny's off-duty
hours, and her sharing of your house; and they can be
avoided simply by switching to a live-out nanny – expensive, but often worth it.

Much worse are the problems caused by employers not
knowing how to treat a nanny with the right mixture of
distance and friendliness. Some – like my fictional wimp
Sarah – are so terrified of telling anyone to do anything
that they end up themselves overworked and resentful.
Others think that a nanny is a slave and – according to
Jane Reed – refuse to consider annual holidays, regular
days off, or paying the legal tax and National Insurance.
So they either become horrible exploitative employers, or
else: they 'Sit around drinking wine every evening with
the nanny until they all get so close that when there's a
problem, after six months, they don't know how to stand
back and get away from it.'

Some are so trusting that they get cheated, or endanger
their children; others go through the nanny's handbag and

diary, until she gets furious and leaves. 'Some of our girls', said Jane Reed in our rueful conversation, 'put hairs or Sellotape across their room doors to trap the employers snooping.' I think someone should set up an Ombudsnanny service, dedicated to mediating in delicate disputes, and dealing with all the seething, unspoken resentments.

In other words, just at the time of your life when you are learning to relate to one quirky, vulnerable, mysterious new human being in a relationship with you you have never experienced before – if you hire a nanny, or *au pair*, you are going to have to work at another new and unprecedented relationship. Your hormones are in uproar, you are only just finding out what sort of a family you are – and you have to adapt to a young woman from perhaps an utterly different region, background and culture. Don't go thinking it's easy. It's possible though, and can be a great enrichment and the foundation of a lifelong friendship. Just to reassure you, let me tell you that our last nanny has now, 15 years later, returned to us as my PA: and that some of our neighbours still have a warm visiting relationship with their Dutch *au pair* from the late 1970s. It can be done.

Things which help: writing down a job description, with hours, duties and yes, overtime rates; having a monthly formal chat about how things are going; and being absolutely clear about what you expect. Ironing adult clothes? Hoovering? If there's an emergency and she does short-notice overtime, will you pay it at a higher rate? Or offer time off in lieu? And can she choose which?

Interviewing is difficult. Choose someone who wants to talk to the child as much as, or more than, she wants to

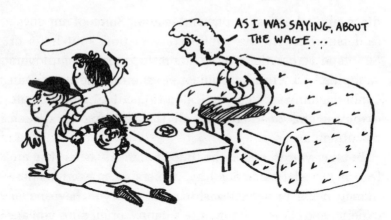

talk to you. The peerless Virginia was down on the floor playing with Duplo bricks before I could even start discussing hours. Note what questions the candidate asks you (if they are all about spare-time use of the car, it is possible that childcare is not her first priority in life …).

Take paper qualifications with a pinch of salt. A newly qualified NNEB may know the correct way to lay out babies' bath equipment right down to the orange-sticks, but may not be all that good with actual babies. You may flinch a little when shown the college 'project book' she has compiled on 'Games to Play with Babies' and find the first ten pages consist of a detailed breakdown, with pictures, on how to play peek-a-boo. Myself, I prefer to find a girl who plays peek-a-boo by instinct.

If you get a casual personal recommendation through a friend, it can be most valuable. A woman journalist, who always seems pretty carefree and unworried to me, has had the same nanny for nine years (and several new babies). 'All I was told was, "She has extremely clean fingernails and she won't run off with the postman." Both true.' If the girl is a complete stranger, read her formal references with great care.

A good tip from Jane Reed is that if you get a very bland reference ('Imogen is a highly experienced nanny who has undertaken the care of my two children,' etc. with never a warm word in it), think carefully. If the last sentence reads, 'I am willing to give a telephone reference and *please do not hesitate to contact me,*' then for heaven's sake, contact them. They may be trying to tell you something awful about Imogen which the laws of libel make them hesitate to type on the reference. Or they may just want to say that there is something odd about her, something which made them uneasy, but they couldn't pin it down ...

If *you* are uncomfortable about anything, ignore all glowing references, even ignore the fact that your children seem to like her. Don't take her on.

Once you have, make her duties clear, her accommodation comfortable, respect her opinions and her privacy, don't abuse her goodwill, and above all, don't vent your own neuroses on her. The worse, the very worst nanny-employers are the mothers racked with guilt about working at all, who hate the fact that their children love and romp with another woman all day, and take it out on her. It should not take much thought to realize what a hellish, downward spiral this will hurl you into. If you start getting that way, give up on nannies and stay at home. If you can afford a nanny's huge wages, frankly, you could afford to come home and mind your own baby. If that sentence outrages you – why then, you are trapped in the childcare rut by circumstance or temperament, and must bite the bullet and not take it out on the nanny.

She's human, after all. She lives with you. Introduce her properly to everyone who comes to the house. Include her in trips and weekends away, if she wants. Oh, and climb down after a row if you happen to be wrong.

One other thing. Talk to mothers with nannies and demanding jobs and you generally find that their greatest dread is the well-liked, comfortable, habituated nanny suddenly upping and leaving, plunging their work and home life into simultaneous chaos. Some nannies know this very well, and use it as a lever to get their own way about everything; but being blackmailed is not pleasant, nor is it necessary. If you have taken care to stay close to your child, he won't have become dangerously dependent. 'When we had one nanny who took to reading the classified ads in *The Lady* in a marked manner at lunch, sighing deeply all the while' say one family, 'we sat down, wrote a letter to a nanny agency and made out a new advertisement for local and national papers, put them all in envelopes, addressed and stamped them, and stuck them in a desk drawer. The letters became a sort of talisman against her stomping out, and made us brave enough to stand up to the more unreasonable demands and complain about the sulking.'

Here, without comment, are some of the answers mothers gave me when I asked what the worst mistakes were which people made in handling their nannies. Some of them are mutually contradictory, but all are useful:

- 'Being too accommodating and ending up doing the clearing away of toys while nanny drinks coffee.'

- 'Giving them a dirty deal, floors to scrub, children to sit up with all night, every night when they're ill.'
- 'Wanting to be liked.'
- 'Boiling with silent resentment.'
- 'Expecting them to be mature and intelligent as well as poorly paid and humble.'
- 'Swanning home from jolly days at work or gallivanting, and expecting to take over and change the pace and mood that the nanny has established.'
- 'Being jealous of the nanny's relationship with the child.'
- 'Expecting someone else to love your child as much as you do.'
- 'Getting muddled about where being an employer ends and a friend begins, and getting to know too much about their private lives.'
- 'Not keeping a day-to-day check on what the nanny is doing. I'm appalled by parents I know who don't see what happens in the child's daily life. The endless tea party/lunch/trip to the zoo syndrome may mean that instead of the one-to-one childcare you're paying for, you have a child who's constantly being ferried around with half a dozen others while the nannies chat. At the end of the day most of us *aren't* selfish cows – some nannies are!'
- 'Expecting your *own* relationship with them to be perfect, forgetting that it's the kids' relationship with them that really counts.'
- 'Not briefing them, ever. Many nannies are very young and like to be told what to do.'
- 'Over-briefing them and giving them too little authority.'

- 'Forgetting that a normal, friendly girl won't want to spend her evenings closeted in a room at the top of the house on her own.'
- 'Not realizing that it is quite normal for toddlers to say they hate people, don't want to see them, etc. just for devilment.'
- Not listening when your child is really telling you something important and alarming about the nanny, because you can't face the awkward truth.

The principles of dealing with nannies also apply to *au pairs* in most respects: but there are important reservations. *Au pairs* work shorter hours, have not necessarily ever *seen* a very young baby before, and expect to live as family. Also, you can't always interview them before they arrive, so many a nervous middle-class family has reluctantly taken delivery of a vast morose Swede, a somewhat pregnant Marseillaise, or a sex-bomb from Hamburg with inch-long fingernails and no intention whatsoever of learning the English for 'no'. *Au pair* horror stories abound, but are easily outweighed by the testimony of families who have found a friend, a helper, almost a daughter. In some ways, the compulsorily 'family' status of *au pairs* is a help; at least you all know what is supposed to happen, and don't teeter awkwardly between being a friend and being an employer. She eats with you, and that is that. 'But anyone', says one long-experienced mother, 'who thinks that an *au pair* is just a cheap nanny, is off their head. She is a different creature entirely, with a different function; and you have to be a different employer. If a trained nanny gets toothache, she gets herself to the dentist at the least inconvenient time possible, and probably even organizes her own substitute while she's away. If an *au pair* gets toothache, you go with her, interpret for her, put her to bed with a whisky toddy, and make a long-distance call to Stockholm to her boyfriend before setting out to collect her English-language homework from her college and buy her some new nail varnish to cheer her up.'

Having a paid helper, nanny or *au pair* can be a happy and friendly experience. There have been times, though, when having made half a dozen of the above mistakes and misjudgements, my only wry consolation was my mother's apocryphal tale of the family who, being fervent Catholics, offered up a sung Mass of Thanksgiving on the day that the children were big enough to let the last, the very last, living-in help depart forever. I suppose they would have had to commission a special prayer for the occasion. And comb the Bible for suitable readings: perhaps Proverbs 5:3 would do:

For the lips of a strange woman drip as an honeycomb,
    and her mouth is smoother than oil:
But her end is bitter as wormwood,
    sharp as a two-edged sword ...

• •

Chapter Eight

Toddlers and
Tornadoes

Years ago, at Oxford, I had a friend with a bushy ginger beard and an erratic temperament. He used to sing 'Carolina Moon' out of his bedroom window through a megaphone, and go on massive benders during which he would insult everybody he knew and then burst into tears. He was fond of me, and at times angelic – amusing, good company, full of Irish songs. At other times, he would swear at me in the street and ruin my dinner parties by attacking people. He went to the Young Liberal conference at Brighton one year, and bought 45 different china pigs because they reminded him of me. He ranged them all on his mantelpiece; it was very touching. One night after a tiff with his girlfriend, he broke into my college and loomed at the foot of my bed in the small hours, accompanied by a horribly drunk Young Conservative with whom he had been having an argument. They wanted to give me a glass of champagne, but had broken the bottle on the way over the Dean's garden wall. Both were huge lads, but one sharp word from me (as I gathered the bedclothes modestly around my shoulders) and they both ambled off home like lambs. In the morning, Guy was contrite; but a little later on he decided that I had somehow insulted him, and smashed every one of the 45 china pigs with a hammer.

I thought about him a lot, during my first years of motherhood. After the intervening decade, in which my life was filled with the sort of mild-mannered, liberal-minded, cheerful and rational people I have as friends, the memory of his little ways was all I had to prepare me for the experience of living with a child of two years old. The crazy tantrums, the charm, the ferocity turning to laughter and back to spite again, the unpredictability, illogical behaviour, and general lovable appallingness of the toddler is reproduced in only a few adults, or even adolescents. If you have mixed with calm and sensible people for many years, you are seriously unprepared for the demon your nice little baby is going to become for a while. All parents would benefit from a crash course to prepare them for dealing with these volatile little creatures. It would help, for instance, to have lived with Dylan Thomas in his wildest period, or chaperoned a fading Sicilian primadonna on her fifth farewell tour, or worked in the private office of an unhinged Fleet Street tycoon. If you could arrange to be the personal manager of a drug-crazed Mexican punk rock band for a couple of years, you would get the general idea.

Anything, really, would help if it got you used to dealing with powerful and erratic personalities. Sometimes, at the end of a particularly rough weekend we used to realize that the root of our troubles was simply that one of the children was at that toddler stage when he or she was the most powerful and forceful personality in the family. The rest of us were like Ben Bolt's Alice: who 'wept with

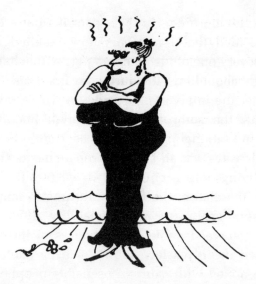

delight when he gave her a smile, and trembled for fear at his frown'. The most high-flying, decisive professionals can be flattened into submission by an even more decisive toddler: I have observed a pair of wealthy, confident business tycoons in a cafe pleading, vainly, with their tiny golden-haired daughter to put her coat on (it was the middle of winter). They lost and slunk away to the BMW with the child still unwrapped. One of our Sunday lunch guests reappeared once, hours after they had driven twenty miles home with their own terrible-two, with a faint desperate query of 'Have you seen a woolly panda anywhere?' We handed it over, and without so much as a cup of coffee, he drove away in a cloud of dust to his distant home, where a small, implacable panda-lover was presumably refusing to go to bed.

Part of the bond between parents of children this age is the way they relate to children's toys and paraphernalia, and stop noticing how hideous a lot of it is. You drop your aesthetic standards in sheer relief at having your children safely and educationally occupied. You forget all the things you used to say about how you'd *never* let a child sit on a potty in the living room, because you're too grateful to him for agreeing to sit on it at all. My own great give-in was over the actual word 'toddler'. I used to hate it; it is Americanese, cutesy and even inaccurate – by the time they stop being big, complaisant babies and become defiant toddlers, most children are walking very firmly and fast, not 'toddling' at all. But alas, no other word describes the phase so clearly; everybody knows what a 'toddler' is, so I have reluctantly begun to use it.

It *is* important to define the phase, if only because there is no point conning yourself that it won't happen in *your* family, and if you expect the worst, whether it lasts two months or twenty, you can only be pleasantly surprised by any let-up. Toddlerhood is the time when the baby, who looked to you for all satisfactions and was pleased when he got them, begins to look into himself as well. He discovers that he has choices, terrible, baffling, enticing vistas of choice: he might go downstairs with you, or he might stay here … he can't decide … he shrieks defiance, because whatever you choose, it is necessary for him to choose otherwise, simply in order to practise the new-found skill of making decisions.

I have carefully avoided crossing a toddler for a whole morning, only to have a terrible scene at lunchtime on the familiar lines of:

'Want orange juice.'

'All right, petal, here it is, lovely orange juice.'

'Want *lemon* juice!'

'Oh, do you? Well, let's put the orange juice away, and here's some lemon –'

'Wanta orange JUICE!'

'There you are, then, here it –'

'DON'T WANT IT! WANT IT! DON'T WANT IT!'

(Hysteria is rising in both of us. I put down both mugs of juice with a gay, forced laugh. He sweeps them both off the table and begins to scream and kick his chair over.)

'MUMMY GO AWAY! DON'T LIKE MUMMY! MUMMY STAY!' Just like a drunk in a Glasgow pub, he wants to fight any Mum in the house, on any pretext.

A psycho-babbling American book described this as 'doing his Independent Person Homework'; you may deplore the language, but you know what he means. Growing babies have to discover their own independence; and the only thing they have to kick against is you.

Further to that, from being a fiddling, casual baby, your child has now discovered that things have uses, and he wants to use them. His skills, however, being limited, he

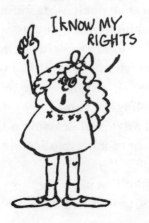

might not manage it first time; his patience being even more limited, he will then throw the toy at you in fury. Well-designed toys allow for this: the Fisher-Price classic gramophone, for instance, has a winder which a younger toddler might not cope with, but that still leaves the on/off switch and the arm to give a sense of control. A badly designed toy, or an older child's toy, may be so frustrating that a tantrum is the only way out. However careful you are, you are bound to run on to the rocks occasionally. When my daughter was born, her 'present' to my son, aged 20 months, was a little wooden tractor. He loved it. He loved it so much that he wanted to sit in it. But it was only 6 inches long. He screamed the hospital down in his rage … but only for a few minutes. After that, he decided to see if the cots rocked, and then to ride in a wheelchair.

With toddlers, you have to go carefully. There is no point shouting at them too early, or at the wrong moment; there is no sense in ignoring the enquiries and overtures they do make, just because you are tired. That little voice at your elbow saying, 'Would 'oo like some soup, Mummy?' and offering an ashtrayful of dog-ends and milk, may not be the most welcome accompaniment to your first sit-down of the day; but if you shout furiously (and unreasonably: who left the ashtray on the low table, anyway? Who showed him how to offer food politely?), you are only aborting a game which – if you had let it develop tactfully – would in fact have given you a happy hour of peace while he played soup-parties and tea-parties with less noxious equipment. If you turn bedtime into a battle, it is you who will have to fight the battle every night. If you force him to eat up his greens, and lose your temper in the process, you are not only making the child unhappy; you are setting up a running conflict which will make you pretty miserable too. For reasons of sheer self-preservation, if no other, you have to be careful and tactful, cheerful and optimistic, when you have a toddler in the house.

If the worst comes to the worst, you can always swear at them. Swearing seems to send all toddlers into fits of uncontrollable giggles, long before they can understand the words. Of course, what will then happen is that they repeat your brief lapses all day long. I speak as one whose innocent child spent the whole of Christmas shouting, 'Oh sod it!' at his horrified granny down from Yorkshire.

The principle is to lead the little rebel through the day by stealth; always making the next step seem attractive, and if possible making it seem like the child's own idea. Develop a habit of offering choices – but never the right ones. If you give a child wide alternatives at this age, he will probably freak out: the enormity of deciding whether to go for a walk or stay at home is too much, at first. But 'Shall we take rabbit or panda upstairs?' 'Would you like a book on the changing-mat?' or 'Is it yellow shampoo or pink shampoo tonight?' are all calculated to cause deep thought while the child, in purely accidental obedience, proceeds up the stairs, on to the changing-mat, and into the bath. If you set out with a firm 'Now then, upstairs for bath-time', with no frills, you are about 60 per cent more likely to hit trouble. On the other hand, offer too many choices and you're stuck halfway up the stairs with an armful of laundry and a child who has changed his mind about rabbit and panda. Play it by ear. Use incentives of a harmless kind to lure him through the day: a favourite record on his way to his nap, a view of a mechanical digger through the kitchen window if he comes for his lunch. If he won't eat, do what all the toddler-books say and try to present his food in a novel way; but don't torture yourself sculpting radishes into hedgehog shapes – there are easier ways. Put it in a grown-up willow-pattern bowl; cut a quick fish shape out of fish fingers. Or sprinkle something on it. At one stage one of mine would eat almost anything provided that the cake-makers' decorations called hundreds and thousands were sprinkled on it. Bacon looked pretty odd, and the same goes for jelly diamonds dotted on a plateful of peas. But it worked, so what the hell.

The other key to heading off terrible behaviour is distraction. I was fascinated by the way a crafty, elderly ex-nanny handled a cross child during a walk on a stony beach. 'Don' wanta come, don' wanta walk, no, want buggy, no, wanta WAAALK.' She just said 'Pish, shush, you're making so much noise I can't hear what the stones are saying. They're talking. I want to hear what they say. Keep your ears open.' The child walked on, stooping, silent at last, fascinated by the squeaking of the pebbles under his sandals. 'If you can't distract a child that young,' said old Janet complacently, 'you're lost.' Another time, my daughter squawked in the car and she said 'Oooh, are you laying an egg? Shall we have it boiled or fried?', and this intriguing thought headed off what might well have been a tantrum.

The crafty toddler-handler makes use of every stage of the child's miraculous, rapid, unfolding intelligence. If you know what rings his bell, you can ring it whenever you like. The speed of progress is fantastic at this stage. Take speech: it seems to go straight from the stage when you are desperately proud of your child's first word, to the point when you wonder, straws in your hair, whether he or she will ever stop chattering all day.

But speech is the key to everything. The earlier a child can talk, properly and clearly, the less frustrating a time you will all have. Once he has the words, he can ask for what he wants, and at last he can point out what he means instead of letting off helpless bellows of rage at the frustrating world.

The stage just before the words come is the hardest of all: a strong-willed baby who cannot make you understand will make you suffer, instead. A grumpy child saying 'Want my milk-lorry' is better than a grumpy baby having an incomprehensible tantrum. Even if the milk-lorry toy is two flights up and you're trying to make lunch. And with speech comes understanding: at last you can say 'in a minute' or 'later'. So if speech develops before mental rebellion sets in, you will have a far easier ride than the other way round: it pays to work for that.

You work on a small child's speech in one simple way: you talk. No point in baby-words; both mine said 'cat' long before they could manage a word like 'pussy'. Clear, repetitive chat gets the message through faster than any tedious attempts to make them imitate you. 'Say "duck" ... go on, "duck",' is in any case a game which palls pretty quickly on you.

Once they can talk a bit, you can start making sure they know the really useful words – like 'dinner', 'drink', 'hot', 'cold' (and eventually 'potty'). Really useful concepts to get into their heads are 'in a minute', 'soon', 'later' and 'one day'. If a baby wants a biscuit and you are halfway through changing another baby, you need the 'in a minute' code to make him realize it is imminent. If you are going out in half an hour, you need 'soon', so that he doesn't throw a tantrum when it isn't 'in a minute'. If Daddy is not home until tea-time, you need 'later'. If the baby wants his own motorbike, you need 'one day'. Saying 'never' is rarely a good idea (except as in: 'Never play with matches' or 'Never hit anybody'). My husband taught me this: he had been in the workshop with Nicholas, who (then just 21 months old) wanted a 'big electric saw'. I said, 'No, you can't have one. No, not next week.' Paul amended this, and averted the tantrum, with 'One day' – a phrase already established as starting pretty far off. On the whole, once there is any under-standing at all and the demands begin, it is worth a bit of effort (and a few silly turns of phrase) to be affirmative more often than negative. If a child asks for a knife, I have trained myself to answer brightly: 'Yes, it is a lovely big knife, isn't it? Sharp, though, so I think it had better go back in the drawer. Yes, one day, when you're 17, you might buy a knife like that.' I sound like a worn old record of Joyce Grenfell addressing her kindergarten class, but it actually works for half the time – which is 50 per cent more peace and harmony than you would have got by saying a straight 'No'. (Still, I wouldn't knock 'No' – you can teach a baby what it means at about nine months, and shouted across a room in emergen-cies, it has saved lives. Just treat it with discretion, that's all.)

When it does come to rules and prohibitions, one thing which seems to help is to appeal to a larger, mysterious world of rules and cause and effect. It takes the heat out of the hand-to-hand battle of wills between the two of you. Thus, 'If *you* go on doing that to Rose, I shall have to take the squirter away,' is a better way of putting it than 'I'll take it away!' It implies an effect rather than a threat. Persuasion to put on shoes, woollies, etc. in winter seems to work better if you bring in some suggestion of universal rules: 'What would people say if you went out with no jumper!' sounds like the utterance of a gnarled old nanny, but let us face it, gnarled old nannies get results. And conversely, it seems to help in a difficult phase if you, the parents, do not pose as the source of all benefits and joys: a child is greatly cheered up if his toy puffin 'brings' him a tangerine, or some mysterious fairy leaves something nice under the bed; it encourages belief in a benevolent universe, which is no bad thing.

Also, a slight atmosphere of conspiratorial mischief between yourself and the toddler does no harm. For weeks my son's favourite game was 'frightening' – running up to people with some object (generally quite neutral, like a teaspoon) and holding it out menacingly at them. Whereupon the victim was supposed to flinch away in terror, crying, 'Oh no! Frightened!' and he would stalk off, quivering with delight. I must admit that I taught him this game (frightening Daddy with a toy fish) as a deliberate diversion and a source of powerful, influential, macho pride. At the slightest threat of trouble, I could head it off with a whispered suggestion that we go and frighten Granny with a piece of Duplo. When he outgrew this, we moved on to other private pieces of mayhem and standing jokes – every other event in his day could be made to glow with achievement and power by cries of, 'Oh no! He hasn't built a – not a TOWER! Well, just as well he isn't big enough to knock it down! Oh no! He's done it!'

If you do not have a toddler yet, this will all make you

cringe. 'Teaching the child to menace people! Suggesting that he overstep the limits all the time! Shocking! Children are naturally kind and anxious to please adults and live in harmony, it only takes reason and kindness to train them in consideration for others ...' The trouble is that toddlers are *not* yet children, they do *not* automatically want to be 'good', and for months and months they don't even want your approval. Love, yes; approval, no. Reason is largely hopeless. Kindness is essential, but they won't be grateful for it. The worst mistake you can make is to assume that because it is walking and talking, a child is mature and sensible. It is *not*. The nearest I ever came to losing a child (and this is all I shall say about toddlers and safety: vigilance is so absolute a need that it runs through every aspect of every day, and there is not much point detailing it) was one day when I had taken him down to the shop, without the omnipresent reins on, for once, and stooped to put the bags in the car. I let go his hand. He was in a good temper, knew his kerb discipline, and I told him to stay close. But in the few seconds he was free, he dashed behind the car into the middle of a busy, fast road, and ran around giggling. It was a joke. Despite his fluency, his quick mind, his general competence, this child was only two years old, and not to be trusted. His own death or injury was so inconceivable to him as to be irrelevant. It would have been my fault if a car had got him; my fault for briefly misinterpreting his character and development.

The better you know your own child, the easier it is not only to keep him safe, but to coax and conspire and jolly him through the day. At 20 months, for example, you may be able to get a slightly unwilling child out of the bath 'so that we can make the water go *schlurrrrrrrrpgurgle*', and

make gurgling plug noises with him while you deftly dry
his ears. By two-and-a-bit you can appeal to more sophis-
ticated, far-off ideas like 'getting dressed and going downstairs to see if Daddy has made your milk and biscuit'
(mention the milk and biscuit to the younger one, and
he'd want it *before* you dressed him, always a source of
trouble). And by nearly three, you can call on a whole
range of madly advanced reasons like, 'Because you're so
nice and clean now that we can put your new rabbit pyjamas on,' 'Because it's nearly time to watch *Teletubbies*,' or
even, 'Because you're such a good boy for Mummy'
(wouldn't put too much reliance on that one, myself).

As a toddler gets older, you can drop some of the exag-
gerated nonsense and conspiracy, and answer sensible
questions sensibly. Even so, the wildly surreal element
will creep back in: for months one of ours ran round the
kitchen shouting 'I am statchering! I am busy, where's my
statcher, I am statchering.' For years we had no idea what
statchering was, and felt that it was probably none of our
business. The only problem was that we never dared to
throw anything away, even if it was an old broken doll's
leg, just in case it was the statcher.

My doctor once asked, when Nicholas was slightly ill
and feverish, whether there was 'any sign of delirium'. I
found it impossible to tell. When you have a child who
sits bolt upright in bed in the morning and says, 'Mustn't
put Daddy's 'letric saw into the washing machine, must
we?' it is hard to separate delirious ravings from standard
daily conversation.

The growth of a child's imagination is very handy for the
parents. From that first moment when a toddler takes a toy

farmer and puts him into a box, saying 'tractor', a vast new world of amusement opens up before him or her. All you need to do is to take it all dead seriously; if that broken stick on the sofa is the tiller of her boat, for God's sake don't move it while she's still up. I had half a morning's tears because I moved a cushion, unaware that it was a bale of hay at the time. If your child urgently needs a wheel for his car, give him a plastic plate, but don't be offended if he won't take it. If he gets totally happy and absorbed playing in the front seat of the real car, and you have a drive where you can see him clearly in it, then take the keys out and let him play there. If that isn't safe, take the odd half-hour to sit in the front with him, reading a paper. I used to get extremely old-fashioned looks from visitors and neighbours when Nicholas was 18 months old, because even in high summer he refused to play on the grass with his paddling-pool and nice beach ball. Instead, he made a beeline for his one true love, the Land Rover. I would sit beside him by the hour, reading or writing book reviews while he beeped the horn and flashed the lights, and the sun poured down outside. How they did stare. Well, I was seven months pregnant, and had hay fever; he was an obsessive Landy-maniac. We did nobody any harm with our little foible.

Only one other general observation on toddlers: on health. For some reason (possibly because they mix more with other children, possibly because they do what used to be known as 'outgrowing their strength') children around their second birthday seem to be especially prone to virus infections. A virus infection, as far as I can find out, is anything the GP isn't quite sure about, isn't a bit worried about, and has 'seen a lot of cases of, out Peasenhall way' last week. A good GP will see you and the child as often as you want, check all the real danger points (stomach, eyes, ears, throat) and very rarely prescribe anything stronger than Calpol at bedtime. His job is to help you keep your nerve, and make sure the illness isn't a serious one in disguise. Mostly, the children seem to have mild attacks of vomiting and diarrhoea, running noses, slight fevers and the most appalling bad tempers. It is like teething symptoms, all over again. I mention the phenomenon only because it seems to be very common, and because it can rattle you very badly when it goes on and on. Nicholas had a good ten weeks when he was never quite well, and I used to sob to my GP that whereas I used to have a healthy, breastfed, tough little baby I now had an ailing, chronic invalid of a child, like something in a Victorian parlour ballad (although less saintly) – and what had I done wrong? Was he pining away because I had selfishly had another baby? Or was he allergic to the twentieth century? And similar nonsense. Meanwhile, night and day, he was crotchety, ill-humoured, undistractible and cross – partly by toddler nature, partly by slight illness. The doctor suggested we give him a urine sample, an effort which occupied many terrible hours (this is not a moment to potty-train). Life was hell.

He recovered, and, looking around, I noticed that all the other ailing little winter-virus children had recovered too, and their mothers had started to comb their hair again and walk with a spring in their step. It passes. The only advice I could possibly offer is:

- If your GP is not sympathetic, change doctors (ask other mothers for advice).

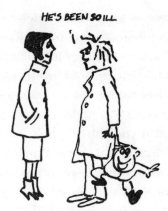

HE'S BEEN SO ILL

- Keep a bag or box of little, intriguing things – whistles and books and balloons and a bubble-tub and sticky pictures – to bring out in desperate moments.
- Keep a jug of orange juice going, fresh if possible.
- If milk is making the child sick, and it normally has milk and cries for it, try substituting honey-water – 1 teaspoonful of honey, a slight squeeze of lemon juice, and hot water, stirred up together. A source of energy and comfort to the tenderest stomach. Have one yourself too, with whisky in it.

Toys and games

Toddlers are, on the whole, mercifully immune to the charms of franchised junk and comic-book spin-off rubbish designed to lure the pocket-money-spending older children. So you can buy your little ones well-designed, educational, durable toys and continue, for a while, to live free from the taint of Spiderman, My Little Pony and Harry Potter spin-offs. It is not only worthwhile, but a positive pleasure to spend money on a few really good, long-lasting multi-purpose toys – like a Fisher-Price farm or a supply of Duplo bricks, and figures which will fit together with the bricks, and later still with Lego. It is also worth touring the jumble sales to see which well-loved, well-used toys still remain functional enough to be sold years later – you would be surprised how small a circle of manufacturers is represented there. And if you actually buy from the jumble sale, even better: no toddler is going to be affronted by getting a third-hand toy telephone, as long as the bell still tinkles.

One slightly tedious task which is also worth doing, for everyone's sake, is a fortnightly (all right, monthly) sort-out of the toys. Get the stacking-rings stacked and the nesting mugs nested if you must; but more importantly, get all the 'cooking' and 'tea-party' things, bought and improvised, into separate baskets, sort out the workbench tools from the 'shop' pieces, and get the constructor-bricks into families (if you are mad enough to have started collecting more than one sort!). This job can only be done, I find, when the children are out of the way; but it does make the toys seem a lot fresher, and less boring, and gives you whole baskets or boxes to lift out while saying firmly, 'Now! We play tea-parties!' instead of groping miserably in a box containing one old shoe, a cup, a dolly's hat, half a Duplo dump-truck and the blade of a toy sword. Similarly, putting things away for a month or two is a brilliant stratagem – between the ages of one and three a child can be given the same extra-surprise-present at least three times, getting bored with it each time after a few weeks and greeting it again with joy after a few more.

I used to dread all this, thinking that to wade through a sea of garish plastic and sort out sordid little dolly-plates was the epitome of dreary maternal slavery. But take heart: you can actually get hooked on it. My monthly Grand Review and Parade of Duplo Vehicles was one of the wonders of the household, lasting all evening while I listened to the play on Radio 4, matching up ladders with fire-engines, and manning various breakdown trucks with the Man in the Blue Hat and Mister Benny Lyn the workman (named, I swear it, by my son. Talk about hypochondriacs).

Making toys is one of the other great unexpected pleasures of parenthood. Making your husband make toys is even better. Since my own husband's penchant for woodwork had been responsible for endless piping infant demands for saws, axes, planes, spokeshaves and plunging-routers, it seemed fair that he should use some of his own tools to make the children their own set. Our toy axe was brilliant, down to the silver paint on the blade: it was cobbled up in half an hour by Paul after I had slogged fruitlessly round the London shops looking for a plastic tomahawk or something like it to fulfil a desperate longing, repeated every morning when Nicholas woke up, for 'My bery own axe to chop logs'. I finally gave up the hunt when a hoity-toity assistant in Selfridge's said, 'Oh no, we do have an Indian suit of course, but no tomahawks, no weapons of violence like that.' All around him gleamed and glistened machine-guns, Death Rays, plastic nuclear-missile-launchers and computer games concerned exclusively with zapping aliens before they even land. And all that my own poor little pacifist had wanted to do was chop wood.

Even if you can't make toys, you can improvise, and, buy, cheap and original things. So I will not speak of the obvious – bricks and carts and suchlike – but pass on oddities from a dozen homes:

- Old typewriters.
- Clothes pegs to fix on the side of a plastic box. ('You find they trap their fingers a few times, then they learn.')
- Shells and stones, selected for unchokeability, to sort out.
- 'Tons of waste paper, felt-tip pens, a plastic tablecloth and a nerve of steel ...'
- A box of old cups (sturdy) and raisins for an instant tea-party.
- The washing-up bowl.
- A supply of old colour supplements to rip up.
- A sheet to fling on a chair for a house, or wrap up in. Better, a very old sheet to rip into strips and dash around with.
- A blunt potato-peeler and a potato.
- Tapes of songs made for small children are popular; but beware. There are some on the market which are merely dreary sub-pop music, on which the children can't even hear the words. Original and clearly sung songs, with funny sound-effects, are in the BBC's *Playschool* and *Play On* series. But be prepared for total addiction. The day the tape with 'Mrs Twisty' on broke, I had the devil of a job getting any cooperation at all for any part of the day. It took three weeks to get another one from BBC Enterprises, during which I was expected to sing this fearful song every day myself, instead. I have never watched the post so closely.

- Florists' solid foam (they will give you the off cuts when they've cut circles from it for arrangements) to break up with a toy hammer. *Not* for chewers.
- Best-ever bath toy: a full-sized decoy duck from a sporting shop. Dick the Duck has spent a whole year in our bath, and between his jolly mallard plumage and his intriguing ability to 'do a wee' (out of the ballast tube underneath) he has given hours of pleasure.
- Old castors. Don't ask me why. Ditto old curtain tassels.
- Ping-pong balls. An amazing range of uses.
- In the garden: just after I spent £30 on a moulded plastic sandpit, some friends bought an old tractor tyre for a fiver, cut the middle out with a bread knife, and made a superb, far safer, nicer one. It has to be the kind of tyre with no sharp wire in it, though. Car tyres are not usually suitable.
- If you can buy an old dinghy that no longer floats, for a fiver (or get one free) it is the best garden present for a toddler whose imagination is developing. Put a mast and cotton sail on, and it beats anything on sale anywhere.
- A safe cupboard full of tins. ('It only takes', says a friend with a notoriously demanding toddler, 'the occasional mutter of "I think I'll have some cat food" to keep him happy for ages.')

But all of these need a bit of a kick-start from Mummy, however little she may feel like playing. A few minutes with the child can lead to a happy half-hour while you get on with everything else; but not always. When I asked one highly skilled father (a lawyer, as you will see) what games a two-year-old was capable of playing without help

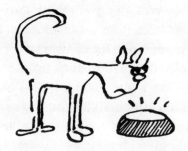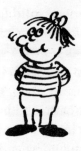

from anybody, he replied: 'Criminal damage, sabotage, apparent suicide attempts, aggravated burglary of the cat's bowl, and uncalled-for manic laughter.' When I asked an even more skilled mother, she simply replied: 'Masturbation'. Oh dear.

But before we leave the subject of toys, I would say that the one thing you *really* can't do without is, for the over-twos, a trike or a sit-on toy to push with their feet. Absolutely nothing replaces it. All the toddlers I have ever known have had long periods of trike pottering, pretending to go everywhere on earth, running bizarre errands 'to get some statchers' or simply sitting, thinking.

Toy control

As time goes on, whatever your resolutions, the sea of coloured plastic will threaten to take over the house. Easy solutions are:

- Have a monthly sweep and put things away if they aren't popular.
- Wicker baskets. ('So inoffensive,' says a user, 'and so easy to aim into from the other end of the room.') One per room.

- Coloured string bags 'hanging, like stuffed haggises, on the back of every single door'.
- 'Ruthless chucking-out of all incomplete or broken toys,' say several mothers, heartily. Easy to say. Suppose that plastic puppy's tail with a burst balloon jammed down it turns out to be the Statcher itself?
- Devote the bottom of a cupboard in each room, kitchen included, to being a glory-hole. At the end of the day, you can sweep every toy inside, shut the doors, and have an adult dwelling again. Wonderful for morale. At the back of the glory-hole you will find your camera, American Express card, powder compact, glasses, diary …
- Trikes and sit-on toys are huge and unwieldy. I know one household where each has a rope strop fixed permanently to the handlebars, and is hung on a Scotch Airer and hoisted to the ceiling at night. You eat dinner with three trikes and a bus dangling perilously over your head, but at least you don't fall over anything.

Clothes for toddlers

Tastes vary. As far as I am concerned, the only healthily selfish rule for mothers of under-threes is never, ever to take them to a clothes shop with you. Take a tape-measure instead. Tape-measures do not get bored and run around pushing things over. Tape-measures do not tip up strange children's buggies and leave the occupant howling feet-up in a binful of bargain socks.

Useful garments which may not have occurred to you are one-piece breathable-nylon (or 'Corfam') boiler-suits which – without being stiff raingear – enable even crawlers and rollers to be out on wet grass or sand without ruining

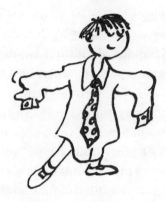

the clothes underneath; balaclava helmets for those who take their hats off in winter; and (says very stylish Nikki Freud) 'Older children's clothes'. They can look very good, she claims. 'Different, but good.' Very Armani ...

Potty training

'Don't do it,' said a canny mother. 'You don't know how easy nappies are until they're out of them, and demanding a poo every five minutes in the shops.' There is something to be said for this point of view. The half-trained baby is a royal pain in the neck, especially away from home and threatening other people's carpets. There is nothing less comfortable than to be constantly asking, 'Do you want to go? Are you sure? Shall we just try?' to the exclusion of all rational conversation with children or adult friends. Even worse, for the adult, is the hawk-like vigilance, watching for signs of knee-clenching, crotch-grabbing or redness in the face of your playing baby. Sometimes you would think the poor little things no longer did anything interesting above waist level; yet if you lapse, it's puddle time. I got back once from the garden to find a shamefaced husband

saying, 'Sorry, I forgot to ask him, we were looking at the house-martins' nest together.' Despite the sopping trousers, socks and shoes, I couldn't blame either of them: baby birds are genuinely more interesting than potties.

Since all this cliff-hanging uncertainty tends to go with early potty training (before two years old) a lot of people go along with my 'Don't do it' friend. Another way of putting the theory of late training was: 'Most of them will be OK by two and a half. So if you start at one, you've got a year and a half of uncertainty. Start at two, and you've got six months. Start at two and a half, and you've only got a week to suffer.' That girl's eldest child, I should say, trained himself at two and a half during a twelve-hour flight to America. 'On an aeroplane 6000 feet up for twelve hours, there isn't much to do except take a child to the loo every twenty minutes.'

Certainly at two and a half most children have realized what is happening, and got a bit of control over it. (You can, though, inadvertently slow this process down by keeping them in highly absorbent, beautifully comfortable nappies, day and night – so well do one-way liners work, so nicely shaped and lightweight is the modern nappy, that a small wee goes totally unregarded. It often isn't until you nerve yourselves to take them off and face the consequences that children – especially boys – actually realize what is going on down there.

However, the pressures to start training early are considerable. Because washing-machines and disposables are such modern phenomena, in your Granny's living memory poor little babies were routinely 'held out' over the pot at a few weeks old, in the hope that a bowel motion might be stimulated by the cold china rim of the pot. Whatever Freud might have said about the traumas set up by early pot training, it was very widespread. (I take great joy from the fact that Jill Freud, wife of the great and gloomy psychologist's own grandson, started training all of hers, she says 'on day 3. Very anti-Freudian. I suppose I am out of step, now.')

Although modern experts on childcare are unanimous in saying that training is pointless under a year, even under 18 months, because the child can't control the right muscles, the old beliefs still hang around to haunt us. 'Oh dear, he shouldn't be wallowing in his own stools at this age ...' 'Shall Granny buy you a nice big potty?' Then friends with trained children come around, leading in their slim-hipped progeny like champion racehorses to shame your baggy-bottomed little recidivist. And then your toddler becomes articulate, and intelligent. There is something almost indecent about an urbane, miniature adult watching you pack up for a morning out with: 'Better not forget the zinc-castor-oil cream, Mummy, in case I do a whiffy. Do I need a clean nappy now, might have done a wee, mightn't we? Have you got the changing-mat handy?' and so on. If he can discuss it so fully, surely he can ... no, he can't.

For it is not always easy to make the penny drop. Some babies actually hate pots, and feel insecure and chilly on them. Some like to go almost immediately on the lavatory, perhaps with a mini-seat, perhaps held. Some (boys especially) have their first breakthrough by going outdoors, behind a hedge. The cardinal rules I gathered from my panel of fellow-suffering mothers were:

- Start in summer, even if your child is possibly too young or too old. Nothing works better than just mooching around in nothing or light towelling pants, letting puddles happen all over the garden until the penny drops.
- 'Trainer pants' of terry backed with plastic are in theory a splendid notion; but if your child hates them, they'll put him off the whole idea. They are certainly hot, rather stiff, and the legs are often too tight.
- The 'peeing doll' technique actually works, especially with girls who can't see anything happening on themselves!
- Once they know what they're doing, there is nothing wrong with incentives. Getting one Smartie each time is not going to ruin their teeth (and if, at this age, you've got them used to having more than one Smartie at a time, you are not too smart yourself). Indeed, one woman, asked how she did it, said airily, 'I sent them to my mother for a whole week and she did it by bribery.'
- Don't automatically assume that bowels will be trained before bladders. All the baby-books work this way, but a few babies refuse to do poos on a pot until much later. Weird, but there it is.
- Never get cross about wet pants. It is counterproductive.
- 'Oh, and do not', said a mother of older children with feeling, 'continually inflict this less-than-thrilling topic on childless visitors.' I thought I would never do this, but after a week or so heard myself babbling on about it everywhere. Mind you, if you have the sort of childless friends who talk boringly about their sex lives or their

operations, I don't see why you shouldn't retaliate. Potty training is really very interesting; why, my children … no, really, did yours do that too? On the sofa? …

- Ignore all grannies (unless they are prepared to take the child home for a week and bribe it).

Away from home

Some enterprising firm recently came up with the potty-training travellers' friend: an inflatable pot. How brilliant! How user-friendly! But certain questions remain unanswered – like how long does it take to blow it up in an emergency and who fancies putting it to their lips anyway, after the first time? Back to the drawing-board, chaps. But the problem of what to do when out with a half-trained or newly trained child with a low-capacity bladder is a considerable one. Canvassing opinion, I came across a large, militant body who believe in using the gutter in emergencies 'and to hell with anyone who stares – they're generally out exercising Great Danes, anyway. Talk about the pot calling the kettle black.' A further militant group points out that 'Every shop has a staff toilet. If they aren't helpful, train your child to stand in the middle of the shop and shout "Poo coming, Mummy!" That'll shift them.' And a small, contented, boy-owning minority said, 'Just take an old cream pot with you and empty the contents secretly down the drain.'

On a car seat, peace of mind can be achieved by laying down two cheap, unshaped but highly absorbent disposables with a terry nappy on top.

One highly organized friend extended this principle by stuffing disposables into a terry-towelling envelope, taking it on buses and out to tea as the child's 'very own special cushion'. She did have a slight problem in discontinuing it once the child was safely trained, but the principle was good. Her daughter never really understood the purpose of the 'cushion', so went on trying to remember to ask for a pot; and the mother knew that so long as the child was sitting at table or on the bus, she was safe from public embarrassment. (Actually, she was in greater danger of this than most of us – her daughter, at two years old, was so tall and so bright that everyone thought she was at least four – which is another common reason for desperate attempts at early training. A four-year-old in nappies looks a bit daft, sideways on.)

Tears and tantrums

The more articulate and clever a child becomes, the more infuriating are its tantrums. 'Unreason, cloak'd in reason's garb', just about sums it up. My son stood by a swimming-pool once, refusing to get off the only dry towel while his nanny and I were shivering and politely asking him to move ('Never force a toddler if you can help it, respect his dignity and autonomy ...' Ah, the old ideals ...). Red-faced, furious, stamping, the little figure clutched the towel and shouted: 'VIRGINIA SHADDN'T HAVE IT! VIRGINIA SHALL BE WET!' (And she was.) Then he tried to stamp on his sister's head. Then he cried and flung himself to the ground as if we had been beating him.

A tantrum, I suppose, is any fit of tears and screaming for which you can't see a reasonable explanation. Nobody accuses a child of 'tantrums' if he yells in fear at an attacking dog, or pain at a fall, or resentment at being trapped in

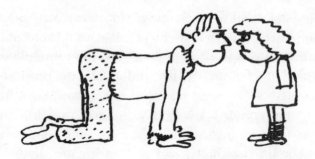

an accident. The trouble is that during the primadonna, Dylan-Thomas-on-the-bottle, lunatic-toddler stage, children treat every small setback as if it were a combination of being chased by wolves and chained in a cellar. There are two schools of thought about tantrums. One, led by Penelope Leach, says that you should get down to the child's level and hold him in your arms safely until it subsides. The other, led by a certain bluff Australian paediatrician, advocates shutting him in his room until the rage is played out. The first system is based on the fact that children can frighten themselves with the intensity of their rage, and need love more than anything else. The second is based on the equally true fact that parents also get frustrated and tense when a tantrum blows up, and need a cooling-off period themselves. Furthermore, where an older toddler is concerned, the lack of an audience often aborts the whole thing much quicker. Certainly the worst possible treatment is a roomful of concerned people, all offering bribes, sweeties, distractions, admonitions and threats in a cacophonous chorus.

But I wouldn't go along with anyone's system too rigidly, if I were you. As with the business of leaving children, you just have to know your own toddler as well as possible, and empathize as far as you dare. Don't let the rage happen, if you can stop it – pay attention to the whining little voice as it builds up. Joke him out of it if you can, quite early on. The following words, uttered loudly and deliberately, have before now turned a volatile child's anger into helpless giggles:

'Don't be OBSTREPEROUS!'
'Shut up, CHICKABIDDY!'
'You little WRRRRETCH!'
'Who's a RAVING RATBAG, then?'
'You little CURMUDGEON!'

That might win you time to create a distraction. Some children can be stopped with a firm 'STOP IT!' but generally not until they are old enough – nearly three – to know precisely what they are doing. Younger toddlers are creatures of pure emotion, and need heading off into laughter, or a new interest. I am sorry to say that even physical force is effective – not smacking (doesn't work) but just picking them up and bearing them off at speed, rocking and whirling and tickling them into hysteria. That this should work destroys all my pet theories about 'children being amenable to reason and having their own dignity which must always be respected'; but in small doses, it cures incipient tantrums like a dream.

A ploy which helped a good deal in our most critical stage was – before the real fury developed – to get the child to *delegate* the tantrum to one of his toys. We have a long-limbed, floppy, skew-whiff rabbit which is ideal. What I used to do was flail its arms and legs around, shouting in a high, furious voice, 'Don't want it, don't like it, don't want it, waaaaaah!' Each child in turn was enchanted at this proof that others suffered the same attacks as they did, and rapidly learned to say, in a low, growling, admonitory tone, 'Rabbit! Bee-have you-self!' Thereafter, we would look anxiously around when the whingeing or shouting began, pretending to believe it was Rabbit. About half the time, the enraged child fell in with this and went happily off to shake hell out of Rabbit.

If the rage develops, here are some treatments (again, many mutually contradictory, but all tested) which mothers have used. At the right moment, with the right child, they all bring peace:

- 'Don't recognize or admit that a tantrum is going on.'
- 'Mimic them, make them laugh!'
- 'Up into the cot, before they can draw another breath – no audience means no tantrum.'
- 'Get down to their level – eye-to-eye works best.'
- 'Change the venue – out quick, to see the ducks.'
- 'We have a large box of coloured buttons and just take them out of the box one by one, slowly, until the child gets interested enough to play with them.'
- 'Be calm, sympathetic, and don't give in. Talking on calmly as though the ear-splitting row did not exist was quite effective.'
- 'Pick them up sharply and go to the cloakroom' (this from a teacher), 'and turn on lots of taps – running water competes with tears and screams.'
- 'Do something "contrary" to shock the curious mind. Put a cushion on your head. Or squeak like a mouse.'

- 'Shout along' (this from a father), 'throw the baby over your shoulder and run. Some babies won't yell or move when carried; this is a primitive instinct.'
- 'Cackle with awful laughter.' (Beware, this offends older toddlers mortally!)
- 'Walk firmly away.'
- 'Sit next to them with a bottle and a chocolate biscuit, both of which will be refused with howls of rage and derision if you actually offer them, but will be shyly and tearfully picked up after ten to fifteen minutes.'
- 'Run around singing at the top of your voice and jump up and down. They get so surprised, they forget.'
- 'Say, "There's another scream coming – I can see it coming out of your forehead, quick, let's look in the mirror and see it coming out, oh dear, it seems to have gone, try again, give me another scream and we'll watch it …"'
- 'Lay them on the floor away from harm then wait, a few feet away. As soon as the noise is over, move in fast and reassure them you love them.'
- 'Say, "You can come back in when you're civilized," and shut them out of the room' (older toddlers only, and only when you can hear and see what awful thing they do outside).
- 'Never, never, never give in. Firmly ignore rigid person and place it out of your sight until screaming stops.'
- 'Sit on the floor, hold her tight, and blow gently into her ear.'

I have tried this last one. I can show you the bite-marks on my shoulder, if you like. Good luck.

Something which helps me to keep my own temper is a chance remark once made by Clement Freud, father of five, years ago when his were all small. 'They're so *brave,*' he said admiringly. 'We're bigger and stronger than they are by far, but look how those little creatures just stand there, defying us.' If for a moment you can see yourself as Goliath with the knotted little features of David looking up at you in defiance, you will be able to muster the love and patience you need not to hit him.

But above all, the thing to remember is that toddlers are not adult people. So afterwards, they won't be embarrassed, or hold anything against you or against themselves. The sun comes out very fast; you have to learn to match their speed of recovery, and pretend it never happened. One day, you'll reach bedtime and realize that it never has.

Bedtime

With luck, this merely continues the tranquil pattern you set with your big baby. Rituals grow more elaborate, even to the point of becoming treats. We used to light candles in the sitting-room and let our son blow them out, or try to: he looked forward to it all evening.

The thing to abandon absolutely is the notion that bed means instant sleep. So long as they're up there, safe and happy, it is entirely their business whether they sleep or not. Often, I would sit writing with the baby alarm at my side, and my two would be gurgling and shrieking at each other and incoherently discussing cats and tea-parties a full hour after being put to bed. I just told myself that this represents the 'quiet winding down' period which every single book recommends having before bedtime, and which we somehow never achieved. Instead, they had a noisy bouncing-around time, and we had a final session of hurling soft animals into the cots while they rolled about giggling; then they could wind down privately. It may not be everybody's way, but it is a perfectly reasonable one. I know of another two-year-old who falls asleep straight away, sleeps for half an hour, wakes up and carouses for an hour or so with her teddies, then sleeps again. In the early stages of this, her parents treated it as a 'sleep disturbance' and spent evenings thundering up and down stairs in turn trying to 'settle' her. Then one night, the husband said: 'She's not crying, you know. She sounds all right to me.' And they left her alone, and she giggled and sang for an hour, then dozed off. A tuck in late at night, and she slept peacefully till 8.00. And still does.

If you have an accomplished cot-escaper, or a child already in a big bed, the problem of late-evening carousing is a bit harder. One mother with a roaming toddler and no intention of spending her evenings crooning and rocking a perfectly happy child, solved the problem by making the bedroom entirely safe (every plug blocked, window barred, every toy checked, no string or plastic bags) and hanging a noisy warning bell outside the door. Apart from once finding her daughter asleep *under* the bed, blankets and all, having forgotten to get back in, she has had no trouble bar some odd sound-effects and chatter down the baby alarm. (Of course, if you have a younger baby asleep in the same room, an even more stringent check of accessible toys and furniture has to be made. But babies sleep through a remarkable amount of upheaval, especially that created by their siblings.)

Groups

One of the most remarkable trends of recent years has been the crazy proliferation of organized infant activities, even among mothers who don't enrol their children in any formal nursery. At any given moment one of your friends will be taking her two-year-old to kindergarten sing-along, another ferrying her daughter of the same age thirty miles to Suzuki violin classes, a third is on the way to ballet, a fourth to under-fives gym, a fifth to pre-Tai-Chi ('so marvellous for his balance'). It can make you feel pretty inadequate if your own child is burbling incoherently to the cat under the kitchen table, or turning out his Granny's box of cotton reels. It is hard to hold on to the old concept of infancy as playtime, when even the UK government is busy setting up a pre-school curriculum and expecting state nurseries to tick boxes every time a baby attains a 'skill'.

All of this is pretty disheartening to those of us whose toddlers resolutely refuse to let Mummy leave them in any group whatsoever, even for ten minutes. Or whose dear little children wade in with such aggression that they get banned, like drunks from pubs, after two sessions of mayhem and GBH among the other tots.

Not only does the dreaded inter-Mum competitiveness place barbs in your side if your child is ungroupable even at three, but your own beliefs can make you uncomfortable. I actually approved like mad of playgroups and kindergartens and early gym lessons and dancing and Suzuki. But one of my children, at least, didn't. Wouldn't join in. Would dance, build, play, turn somersaults happily at home, or with one familiar little friend, but went rigid when the other children were there. Certainly wouldn't permit some playleader to interfere with his intentions, or knead his playdough. Other families, kind and cultivated and sensible and disciplined households, are shamed at groups when their toddlers turn into monsters of violence when put into a room with a dozen others: they smack, and push, and snatch, and bite as if they had been brought up in the gutter, fighting for scraps.

If either of these things happen to you, all that you can do is stand back for a moment, refuse to compete or compare, and question the accepted wisdom about play-groups and nurseries and formal preschool education in general. Remember that it is quite a new fashion; you could argue that the natural way for a child to develop under five is within a family, close to his parents and siblings, knowing his neighbours and one or two children. You can see by merely watching some children that they are actually happier being one rung of a social ladder – with older children and younger children – than they are among a group of their peers. If you think about it, there is no particular reason why a three-year-old (still less a two-year-old) should want to be with his exact peers. Indeed some of them regard children of the same age with a sort of horror; a sort of, 'What, am I not the only one?' attitude and a sense of fear and threat. Hence, perhaps, some of the violence and the clinging.

If your child doesn't like going to groups, perhaps the group is wrong, not him. Some educationalists are even daring to suggest that children learn more, not less, if they stay at home with their mothers all day. And there are terrible sights at some very expensive and good nurseries; not cruelty, not even physical neglect, but just the sad spectacle of some child who is withdrawn but quiet, and gets ignored in the corner, looking at the wall, because he or she is 'no trouble'. No trouble, but having no fun either, and learning nothing. A child who is not ready for a group should not be dumped in one, unless you are in extremis. A child who wants only his mother should have her.

Which the mothers, of course, may not like one bit! Apart from all the education which the child is supposed to be eagerly gulping in, playgroups and classes provide maybe the first free time for a mother in three long years. Even if you are not trying to work during those hours, other solutions must be found. Some families club together in twos and threes to hire a good babysitter for a couple of mornings a week, who runs a sort of mini-play-group for a close, familiar little group. Supplied with pasting and painting and modelling equipment, and with at least one of the Mums drifting in and out on each of the mornings, this can do everything a playgroup can, on a smaller scale. If you are alone, or broke, you still might organize an exchange of children for a morning or two; even if the other children are quite a lot older. Anything to bridge, for your child and yourself, the gap between exclusive baby-life and adult socializing.

Families on the far side of this dilemma, with children who were slow starters but now trot happily into play-groups and primary schools, advise a few precautions for the final moment of taking the plunge: some or all might work for you.

- Teach them all the songs at home, first. Get the playleader to give them to you.

- Check the activities they will be asked to do, and practise those at home too.
- Send in a familiar flask and cup for the mid-morning snack.
- Never be even a minute late to pick your child up, at first.
- Teach plain and universal words for potties and lavatories. Don't hesitate to take your own pot, even if they have pots there, and label it and tell the playleader. Embarrassing though it may be, when the other children are roaring in and out of strange lavatories like ten-year-olds, it is better than ruining your child's first stab at independence (and *your* first free morning for years) just for the lack of a familiar comfortable rim round a small bottom at moments of need.

Clinging

This is an allied subject, and problem, except that it happens at home too. Again, advisers divide into those who say, 'Leave them to scream, they'll learn that you always come back into the room in a minute,' and those who say, 'Take them with you, even to the lavatory, it will give them confidence.' The insistence of some children on coming into the very lavatory with their mothers is something which recurs again and again in maternal confidences; it is somehow symbolic of the total taking-over of your life. 'I waited ten years,' said one girl dramatically, 'for a private pee!' Others admit to having had toddlers perched on their knee on the lavatory for months. One old-fashioned mother, her children now adult and urbane, said, 'I used to see those four little hands coming under the bathroom door and I wanted to *stamp* on them!' This particular foible seems to bring out a special kind of desperation in all of us.

Which sort of advice to take is a puzzle. Perhaps a bit of both: take them with you often, but occasionally leave them with a repeated incantation of 'Back in a minute'. Get whoever is still in the room with them, if anyone, to say it too. Jump on them sometimes when they're *not* demanding cuddles, and smother them with unwanted hugs and protestations of adoration. It is impossible to tell a child too often at this age that Mummy loves it. For remember, as one mother said, that 'Clinging is love. They are saying their love, crying their love for you.' Even inconvenient love is worth respecting.

Of course, you could always adopt my old system of singing very loudly in the lavatory or the coal-hole or wherever you have gone, so that they know you're still there, just round the corner. 'Shoals of Herring' is a good one, or the Battle Hymn of the Republic.

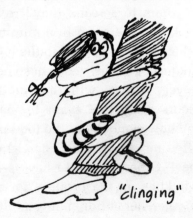

"clinging"

• •

The Second Lap:
Siblings

I was at a Christmas party once, filled with people at our own stage of child-production. A good few pregnant bumps were sailing around, and small children crawled and mountaineered across the chairs and pinched food and tugged furiously at the wrong parents' trousers and skirts, demanding potties. Given a few minutes' leisure to wave a drink and attempt an adult conversation, I found myself in a corner with a young father, similarly let off the hook. We were all contemporaries; we had earnestly discussed birth together, compared midwives, swopped enema stories, argued about breastfeeding, and seen our babies rise to their feet together and push one another off tricycles. We had been through the mill, in company.

I, however, was one of the first pioneers in this set to have risen to the next rung on the ladder. Not only was Nicholas happily fossicking around in a bowl of crisps at one end of the room, but Rose, aged five months, was sitting in a rare fit of silent happiness on her Granny's knee at the other. So the young father, glancing round at his own vastly pregnant wife, asked me the obvious, dangerous question.

'Tell me,' he said. 'What's it *like*, having two of them?'

And I thought for a little while, and remembered the early mornings, the complicated two-stage bathtimes, the unsynchronized feeds, running battles and running noses. I cautiously flexed my shoulder, sprained by carrying two infants upstairs simultaneously. I looked at his carefree, innocent face. And I said, 'I do not think that I had better tell you that.' So we left it there, and two months later he found out anyway.

One common trait of parents with two or more children under five is a sort of exasperation at the complaints and worries of parents with only one. It parallels exactly the sense of amused contempt which the sleepless new mother feels for her pregnant, carefully analytical, hopelessly idealistic friend. Now that I have two myself, I have occasionally glimpsed a flicker of the same contempt in the eyes of friends with three or four children. No doubt mothers of twelve think that we are *all* wimps and weaklings who don't know what Life is all about.

There is no point beating around the bush. A second child changes everything, again, just as life was getting on to an even keel with the first one. Just when you thought it was safe to go back in the water ...

Assuming that you take the popular gap of between one and three years from baby to baby, what happens is this: you have a child getting to its feet, taking walks with you, asking endearing questions about ducks, coming to terms with a pot, inviting you to imaginary tea-parties – and then, suddenly, you are plunged back into the warm, dim world of nappies and helplessness and unpredictable demands. Just as you get used to making bargains ('Five minutes while I get this done, and we'll go to the park to sail your boat') you suddenly have a tiny, implacable Ayatollah who wants feeding NOW! INSTANTLY! before you can even get your buttons undone, let alone finish the playdough model for the elder one. Just as two parents get into a weekend rhythm of giving each other time off by taking the lone child out for an exciting walk, suddenly both parents are needed on duty simultaneously, if one is not to crack up with exhaustion and if the child is not to miss out on exciting baby-free walks. If you are an earning mother, the three-way split (child, work, self and husband) turns into a four-way split (child, other child, work and heaven help yourself and husband). Your style of motherhood may change: if you have never smacked, just wait until the first deliberate, naughty, dangerous attack on the defenceless new baby – and watch your hand swing round involuntarily to slap the marauding toddler. If you have never resorted to bribes, wait for the first time

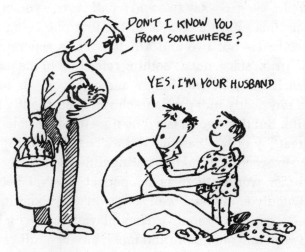

that a breastfeed can only be achieved with the aid of Smarties for big brother. If you despise all the selfish-cow techniques I have offered for getting time to yourself, you may begin to look back at them now – as ways to get a few moments to pay attention to the baby.

You will probably end up singing the Alleluia Chorus and blowing soap-bubbles simultaneously, while sneakily spooning Farex down the baby; because you know that if you stop entertaining the toddler he will get restless, and do terrible things with the rest of the slimy mush while you are coaxing the baby's mouth open.

If you have a very short gap between babies, the elder one mightn't get jealous – a one-year-old finds everything so new that a baby is just another marvel. On the other hand, you will have long periods to endure with two sets of nappies on the go, and be physically stretched to your limit (doctors grumble at women who don't leave more than 18 months between pregnancies). If you have a slightly longer gap – say two and a half years – you may be fitter and may have a chance of the first one being more independent – but two and a half years is generally the peak tantrum stage, not a soothing reflection in the postnatal haze. If you wait even longer, and go beyond three, you have a physically independent, clever, even slightly helpful child. But three years is a long time to be the sole focus and great joy of two parents. It may be difficult, to put it mildly, to accept a wrinkled, boring little rival.

In other words, there is no perfect interval between babies, and you might as well stop worrying about it.

I had a gap of 20 months. They played together a little, after a year, and later more and more; but for a full year we had two sizes of nappies stacked in the bedroom, making morning, evening and naps a non-stop parade of mucky bottoms. And for at least ten months it was a regular thing to have to carry both upstairs together, when the toddler had a fit of regression to babyhood.

His regression, incidentally, was nothing to mine: it is a great unacknowledged shock to the maternal psyche to go into hospital one day still referring to your elder child as 'the baby', and come out days later with another baby holding the title. I had tearful postnatal nightmares in which my real, first baby was snatched away and replaced by this rather dull new version. And when I woke up, there was the first baby, still there, but with enormous size seven feet in huge leather shoes, covering the tiny toes I had once counted. I used to burst into tears at the sight of his feet for weeks, and even a stray shoe on the landing at night could send me off into a storm of weeping. It embarrasses me even to think of this phase now; but I offer it, cringeing slightly, as evidence that second babies change all sorts of things. Mothers easily think of their babies as younger than they are, and the shock of a new sibling can bring it home, with pain, that children grow up and will one day walk away on their huge lumbering feet.

Weeping over shoes, however, is something of a luxury. It fades away as the hard facts of life with children (as opposed to life with one pet child) begin to make themselves felt. To begin with the simple, logistic problems:

Timetables and routines

The comfortable, familiar routine which suits the toddler is quite different from the hippie, freewheeling, unpredictable life of the demand-fed baby. The first few months, frankly, are going to be chaos. The only thing which seems to help (apart from actual help, which may be scarce) is keeping the new baby in the centre of things – in a basket in the kitchen, or somewhere handy in a pram – so that you don't have to keep breaking off games or jobs to tend it. Few things are more frustrating than having a toddler too young to be safely left alone downstairs even for five minutes and having to choose between a sprint to the bedroom for the baby, or a session of persuading, coaxing and final carrying of the older child upstairs to change a nappy there.

Frequent advice to parents of jealous children is to time feeds and baby-worshipping for moments when the older one is having a nap, or out for 20 minutes playing at the neighbour's. It is good enough advice from the children's point of view, but ignores the fact that if the demands of the two babies alternate like this, their mother gets no time at all to breathe freely, eat or sit down alone. This doesn't matter too much if the evenings are free; but very few babies under three or four months are asleep in the evening; and a day which begins at six and ends at eleven or twelve at night is just plain terrible. As far as I was concerned, the breakthrough came when I managed to synchronize the afternoon naps of the two babies. With that hour and a half off, even if it was spent tidying up the chaos of the morning, anything seemed possible.

A very nice routine can develop by six months: in ours the baby had a morning sleep, which gave big brother the prescribed 'private time'; lunch was communal (except that there had to be some particularly amazing delicious pudding to distract him from the baby's sneaky top-up breastfeed); both had a nap sometime between one and three. (Then the whole thing collapsed in chaos around bathtime, but that is another story.)

Transport

If the big one isn't yet a reliable walker, pedestrian expeditions are fraught with perils and irritations. The conventional solutions are:

- Sling-and-buggy. The cheapest. Requires a strong back. I am told that on occasion, 'the older child, held at arms' length while the baby is strapped to your breast, feels that his place has been usurped'. You might have to pick up the toddler, and the buggy, and the shopping, to go down an escalator or solve a tantrum. Think about it.
- Pram with a pram-seat. I know many people who have used this with serenity and confidence. I suppose it depends on the occupant of the pram-seat. My one attempt led to the baby being catapulted in the air several inches as the seat occupant bounced on the amazing, Royal-baby-style super-suspension of the pram. Another friend used it for months and reports: 'A disaster – the times I came out of a shop to find three children in hysterics because it had tipped up!' And as for attempting to use a pram without a pram-seat, another friend reports: 'My husband (after I had told him not to) tried putting my son on the end of the pram, and ended up with a 17-day-old baby lying in the road, so be warned.'

- Double buggy. If you can get the sort which partly reclines, you can use one from about two months. Undoubtedly the best of a bad bunch of options; but choose carefully. Some are built to be no wider than a standard wheelchair, and will therefore go through the doors of most shops. Some are a full 6 inches wider than this, and will not. Some are so heavy (because of fancy pram-bars, everyway tipping mechanisms etc.) that you can barely lift them folded up. All of them are hideous to manoeuvre (especially with a thumping great three-year-old in one side) on pavements and steps. One, an excellent make, 'actually snapped, having had too much pressure put on it when the heavy side was constantly suspended in mid-air while I manoeuvred around prams, people and baskets of shoes displayed on the pavement'. All win dirty looks from passers-by, who seem to consider them an unfair contrivance designed to gouge holes in their ankles. None will be as good on rough tracks as singles. But

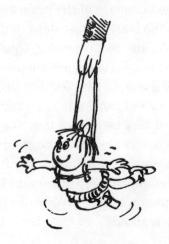

they are comradely; the babies do seem to talk to one another quite early on, and when the toddler wants to walk, you can put the shopping in his seat.

- Reins. Even if you disapprove of walking children on reins, it helps to have a set of lightweight webbing ones on the toddler, for those delicate and critical moments when you are trying to fold the buggy, hold the baby, keep the shopping, and find change for the benighted pay-as-you-enter bus.

Car transport

In the old days, before Road Safety was invented and when a car that did 60 mph was a hotrod, children used to be bundled into the back of cars and clouted if they pulled the driver's hair. In this way, families of six would roar around in Morris-Minors and Hillman Minxes without a thought. Now we all feel rightly guilty – and are wholly illegal – if we allow a child to travel anywhere without a seat or straps. But the arrival of the second, then the third child creates fearful problems. A small car may not be able to accommodate three securely fixed child seats, with a reclining type for the baby, in the back. Babies' recliners should never be in the front, especially if you have an airbag (it's lethal), and in any case the back is safer for all children. Short of buying a huge people-carrier there is not much hope of comfort; and moreover, the bigger child will be able to get at the baby if a malevolent mood comes on. Oh, and the baby, once gripping and tugging enter into his skills, will be able to pull the elder siblings' hair. As one multifarious friend observed, 'I put mine in the middle, she can grab both her brothers' hair at the same time and my driving is punctuated by yells from both of them and great gales of laughter from the baby.'

Jealousy

All of these logistical problems, however, are a matter of management and ingenuity and a bit of money. The great threat which hangs over every family from the moment the second pregnancy makes its dark ring in the test-tube is something which can be solved by none of these things: it is Jealousy. Will the Mk I baby mind the arrival of the Mk II baby? Will it ruin his life? Will the Mk II baby be bashed/neglected/grow up in the shadow of the firstborn? Will they be friends? Terrible old grannies and neighbours say things like, 'Dear me, your nose is going to be put out of joint, young lady, isn't it?' Or, nearly as bad, 'You'll soon have a little brother to play with you, aaah.' (He won't. If he expects a playmate he will be badly let down, for over a year.) Friends tell you tales of elder siblings who have scratched, bruised, mauled or tried to smother the new baby. Even our best baby-book writer, Penelope Leach, compares the child's shock to your coming home and finding that your husband has brought in a new wife and expects you to be friends with her. (Sent me into hysterics, that one did, until commonsense reasserted itself.) A baby is *not* a grown woman, or a wife. The relationship is different; strong, but different. A child is, after all, programmed to know deep down that one day he will strike out without you; the same is not true of a wife, except perhaps in the television saga *Footballers' Wives.*

Some families have no problem at all with sibling jealousy. Fights, yes, later on when the baby actually grabs the

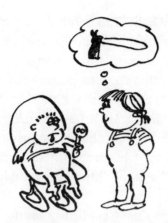

big child's toys; but not that deep, miserable, brooding jealousy of a mother's and a father's attention that we are led to believe is almost inevitable.

'We worked so hard at avoiding it,' says one mother now, 'that the younger one is now jealous of the older one!'

'No problems at all, quite honestly,' says another. 'She loved the baby from day one, the baby was good and quiet and sleepy, and later adored her sister. I got jealous, actually!'

There are, from common experience and often repeated, a few safety precautions worth taking against the green-eyed peril.

- If you tell the toddler there's a baby in your tummy, make him understand that it's his as well.
- Put a present in the cot on his first visit to hospital, 'From the baby'.
- Involve the older brother or sister in the routines of bath and change. ('Oh, a nappy! Thank you!' you cry,

sticking the poor baby into a vast child-size disposable
so as not to hurt the donor's feelings – poor old Rose
could hardly see over the top, sometimes.)
- Make damn sure that tactless visitors to the house don't
coo over the baby and ignore the toddler, and that
uncles and godparents are briefed to bring some tiny
thing for *both* children, if they must bring rattles.
- Fuss and cuddle and admire your beloved eldest and
don't gaze into the baby's blue eyes all day long.

If you do all that, you have set things on the right track.

But whatever you do, jealousy is a fact of life; and a
toddler lives in a permanent whirlwind of uncontrollable
emotions; and he *has* been deposed from his sole-child
status, and he *does* get less private attention than he did,
just at a time when he wants more. There is absolutely no
point in pretending that the problem doesn't exist, least of
all to yourself.

A solid piece of advice comes from Jill Freud, who
brought up five children: 'I don't think that you can stop a
child being jealous if he is, because he *is*, and that's all
there is about it. But I wouldn't hesitate to let him know
that he can't take it out on the baby or bash him – I wouldn't
wait to be tactful any more than I would be tactful about
stopping him running under a car. Good social behaviour
is a fact of life, and he might as well learn it sooner rather
than later. It is easier for him, too.'

This robust attitude has the great advantage of
completely lacking the one complicating factor which
makes maternal treatment of jealousy often so heartbreak-
ingly incompetent (I speak as a frequent incompetent);

and that is our old friend, Guilt. It is actually possible to feel guilty for *having* the second child, and so 'letting down' the first. Then you feel guilty about not loving the second enough ... It is not a spiral to allow yourself to go too far down. Repeat Jill's words like a mantra: 'Good social behaviour is a fact of life, and he might as well learn it sooner rather than later.' Steer clear, for a while, of your acquaintances who have beautifully behaved, affectionate, balanced only-children, and stick to the tearful, tattered company of your own fertile kind.

Here are some ploys for helping children get on together from birth. A lot of them, coupled with blind faith, do work:

- A brand-new baby's greatest talent is staring. If you point out to your playing toddler that the baby is 'looking at you', he will be pleased. He is an exhibitionist. The baby perched safely on a lean-back chair on the kitchen table is out of reach, but can be shown things and shown off to. The elder one may get quite annoyed when the baby looks away: she is his audience and top admirer.
- Its other great talent is sleeping. As far as possible, ignore the baby totally while it is asleep.
- Refer to the baby constantly as 'Nicholas's sister' or 'Arthur, that's Isabelle's little brother' to keep her or him firmly centre stage.
- Get the older child a little pet – a gerbil, a fish, a rabbit – as a diversion from the endless baby-talk in the house.
- 'Grit your teeth,' says a mother of two, 'and cuddle the

older, jealous one for an intolerably long time however daft it may seem.'

- Convince the older child that the baby likes him. Don't suggest that he ought to like the baby; that's irrelevant to him. But if this staring, perhaps now smiling baby smiles at *him,* point it out.
- Once the baby starts swiping and grabbing things, build her/him up as being 'naughty' or 'mischievous'. The first time my son smiled entirely without strain or suspicion at his sister was when she threw a whole mug of milk on the floor and laughed. 'Rose is making a *mess,*' he said, with happy reverence.
- Also point out that the baby will grow bigger, and come under the same disciplines as himself. It is absurdly obvious, but easy to forget, that a two-year-old knows little of time and development; it wasn't until one day mine said, 'Rose might grow into a *proper* baby,' that I realized I'd never told him this. From then on he got constantly told that one day, she too would take on the grave responsibilities of being two, and get shouted at for messing, or being a pest, or whining.
- Keep your visitors under control. It is unforgivable to come into a house and coo over a baby while a lumpish, less attractive toddler with a running nose looks on despondently. Some people manage to get the toddler to show off the baby; seriously jealous children won't be duped this way, and the only thing is to boast of their great achievements to the visitor, if necessary removing the baby forcibly from their cooing, soppy grip. Small babies do not get hurt feelings. Trade on this while you can …

- Praise extravagantly any efforts your child may make to play with the baby. Cooperate tactfully in games. We had a damn-fool game in the bath, in which the baby grabbed a ping-pong ball out of her brother's toy boat, and I shouted 'Who said you could steal that egg?' (There is a favourite book about an egg-stealing fox.) Then I gave it back and the game started again. If I wasn't helping, the game would be a fight. With intervention, it made them both happy.

- Try wilfully misinterpreting your child's intentions. 'Oh, are you bringing Harriet your hammer to look at? How nice, she is pleased. Yes, you pat her on the head, good old Harry, only a silly old baby, but she's all right, isn't she, but you'd better take that hammer away, she's too small for hammers, isn't she …' This has strong comic overtones for onlookers – a cooing, optimistic mother fending off an embittered hammer-attack while pretending it isn't happening – but it is oddly effective. Everyone wants to believe the best of themselves.

- Let the toddler know that you understand. 'The baby is a pest sometimes, isn't she?' can work wonders.

- Putting two cot-bound siblings in the same bedroom can work an overnight miracle. They wake up in the morning, find no adult around to be competitive about, and fall back on each other for company. At last the toddler has an audience for his repertoire of squeaks, thumps and tuneless renderings of 'Goosey Goosey Gander'.

But above all, CONTROL VIOLENCE. A child who has made a baby cry is not really pleased; he is miserable. The further you let the violence go (a real bash as against a threat), the worse the whole situation gets, now and for months to come. Ways of controlling violence are:

- Having a baby doll around for the child to bash instead. I dislike this; many swear by it.
- Never leave them together, even for a moment, out of your sight until you really know they will be all right.
- Let it be clearly known that if the crawling baby approaches the toddler's toys or buildings with intent to cause malicious damage (which is all the time) he has only to call you and you will remove the baby. If you fail to keep this promise, you risk retaliation falling on the bald little head of the invader. But it is difficult to punish a child who has just had a huge Lego castle demolished.
- Have a firm rule that if the baby (or anyone) gets hit with any weapon, or any toy used as a weapon, that object will be *taken away* and not seen again that day. I rigorously applied this rule from the day of the first irritated swipe with a beloved plastic spanner, and it works; the taking-away rule applies even to semi-accidental blows. The point of it is that the damage a child can do with his hands is limited. The damage he or she can do with a weapon hardly bears thinking about. And I say 'he or she' in this case advisedly: it is a fatal mistake to think that girls' natural maternal instincts will prevent them from being violent if crossed.

I have (although this is tricky ground; diplomatically) also taken weapon-toys off visiting children who bashed mine; and naturally, any rattle the baby poked exuberantly in a larger person's eye got removed with exactly the same show of ceremonial rule enforcement.

- Finally, whatever you do, keep emotion out of it. The force of your protective maternal rage (even if you secretly still rather prefer the toddler) can take you by surprise. But furious defence of the baby only upsets everyone. Try not to think like a tigress defending her cub. Think like a slightly bored, very experienced, basically kindly policeman outside a football ground.

Besides, if you keep emotion out of it your brain can continue to work. And as one mother was taught by a gentle Mexican *au pair,* and passed on to me: 'Confrontation with a small child is a sad and unnecessary business. The mother is stronger and cleverer and can always find a way round.' And should do, not least when it is a question of meeting a demand, however violent and perverse, for something as simple as love.

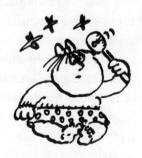

• •

Chapter Ten

High Days
and Holidays

A great truth came to me once, in a punt. There were seven
of us aboard: one husband, punting; two mothers, each with
an eight-week-old baby strapped to her chest; and a boy and
a girl, each about twenty-two months old, and each attached
to its mother's wrist by a set of reins. The reins were
stretched bar-taut as the toddlers hung out over the side,
looking for crabs. We mothers, hanging on like grim death,
tried at the same time to avoid sudden movements which
might wake the sleeping babies in their slings. The husband
(hers) punted doggedly on through the mud of Thorpeness
Meare, dreaming a little wistfully of the old days on the
River Cam, when there were strawberries and champagne
instead of rusks and Ribena, and the girls leaned back seduc-
tively in wispy white summer dresses, instead of hunching
anxiously over babies and smelling of stale milk.

Three things happened, then. The toddlers simultaneously got fed up with looking for crabs, and began to tug
violently at their harnesses. The two babies woke up and
started crying. And it began to rain. With that grim,
resigned maternal persistence which has kept the human

race going for a million years, we unbuttoned our blouses and began to feed, the rain dripping down our cleavages. We pulled waterproof hoods over the four downy heads of the children, but let the drizzle fall unimpeded on our own lank hair. Michael punted stickily towards the shore, looking warily around in case he should be recognized while in charge of this fearful menagerie. Somewhere, a golfer on the banks shouted 'FORE!' and ribald remarks were made about our four bouncing breasts.

And at some point, one of us (I forget which) said, 'Well, this is nice,' and the others agreed, without irony. 'Yes, isn't it lovely to be out.' And it was then that the great truth came to me: the great knack of being a parent of small children is to *lower your expectations* of ordinary adult pleasure. If we had looked at it another way, we were having an absolutely dreadful time, soaked by the rain, immobilized by the babies, tormented by the toddlers, able to converse only in snatches. But the way we saw it, we were doing splendidly: none of the children was crying, all of them were perfectly safe, we had a change of scene from our kitchens, and the chance of a few ribald adult jokes about golfers and boobs.

It hardly seemed to matter, with all those tiny victories piled up in one morning, that a suspicious smell was rising by now from at least three of the four nappies in the punt. We climbed damply ashore and set off home, rejoicing in the knowledge that the toddlers were thoroughly tired out, and would sleep after lunch while we read the Sunday papers. Small, significant pleasures.

You have to grab at the small pleasures, especially once you have two or more under-fives. You have to expect the worst, and be resigned to never again leaving a teashop, or a boat, or a weekend cottage with dignity (it always seemed to resemble Napoleon's Retreat from Moscow by the time we reached the door; either one baby or the other would be shrieking with fury because it didn't want to leave, or else shrieking because it *did* want to). You have to prepare for an expedition to the seaside as if you were kitting out a space mission, and be philosophical about it if the child hates it all when you get there. I used to be openly contemptuous of parents who just stayed put at home for five years, or went only on expeditions designed exclusively for the children; but I grew to see their point. Without great determination and lowish expectations of pleasure, attempting adult pastimes with small children in tow can seem to be barely worth the trouble. Indeed, I have sometimes thought that the one thing you should never try to do is to go, encumbered with small children, on the sort of expedition you most fondly remember from your single days. We have sat on our boat, on a fine breezy day, with one baby being sick and the other having a toddler scream-up about his safety harness, and thought that it would be a million times better not to tantalize oneself with old, free, wild memories of real sailing.

People do keep up their bachelor pursuits, though; I know a woman racing driver who took her baby along (and made him special earplugs to shut out the noise of the track).

Yachtsmen strap babies into bunks, and tether toddlers on deck with a bucket of stones to play with as they swish along in a brisk and chilly Force 7; small figures in buggies look out wonderingly at greyhound tracks, at tennis matches, at miniature hovercraft rallies and county shows. In the case of activity sports, I have seen one parent hang-gliding while the other minded the children on the ground, waiting to swop places; watched little babies craning up at Mummy on her big parachute; and (on a more mundane level) seen parents taking turns to swim lengths in the big pool while the other one splashes with the orange-armband set in the paddling trough. It can work, with a bit of determination, a lot of organization, and (here is the crunch, too often) the cooperation of both parents.

Because you *need* two guardians if anybody is to enjoy an adult amusement in the company of small children. Mummy taking the children to watch Daddy play cricket is all very well, but (unless Mummy is a really passionate cricket fan) it is not much more than a change of nursery scene, for her. She, and the children, might be better off in the park, just meeting the sweating and victorious Daddy for tea. On the other hand, if you both get a crack at the sport, or spectacle, or whatever, and both take a turn with the mewling babies, *both* go home feeling victorious. (There have to be moments, of course, in any marriage when resentments boil up to a nice healthy stew: I reckon that my worst attack came when I sat beside the car, in the dust, outside the Royal stables at Sandringham spooning cold mutton-and-barley dinner down a seven-month-old baby in a heatwave, while Paul strolled about inside discussing the fine points of carriage-horses with the Duke's grooms. However, I later swanned off to row up the Thames while he fielded a teething baby and a toddler fighting-drunk on Calpol, both noses running solidly for two days. I think I got even.)

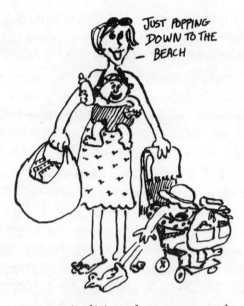

To come to practicalities: there seem to be two essentials for incorporating babies and small children in expeditions: preparation and timetables. Preparation is obvious; if you set out in a car without nappies, wipes, cream, spout-mugs, juice, damp cloths, dry clothes, empty plastic bags for nameless horrors to be sealed up in, toys, buggies, sunhats or winter hats, etc., etc., you risk all manner of irritations. A bit less obvious is the need for rigorous timetables; if, for instance, you have a baby who gets fractious without an after-breakfast nap, then you need to make sure there is a decent car ride or uninterrupted sit-in-the-buggy for that hour. If you have children who go off at the deep end without a 12.15 lunch, then you need either to be somewhere nourishing at 12.15, or to carry a lot of biscuits and fruit around. And if you have a toddler who dislikes being in the car at all, then the worst thing you can do is strap him in, rush back into the house for something, try to hurry up a dilatory partner, get involved in a telephone conversation, and delay the whole trip a quarter of an hour. The toddler will start fractious and continue fractious.

It is sometimes the timetable aspect of family outings that totally discourages either father or mother from attempting them; if you have spent your youth making spur-of-the-moment plans, staying out late without notice, dropping in to pubs on impulse and eating at odd hours, then small children come as a bit of a shock. Frequent wailing arguments may be heard, on balmy Bank Holidays, between couples in which one parent has imperfectly understood the principle of infant outings:

'We're not running a bloody railway timetable! I want to see the next race!'

'Yes, but what do you think will happen if Debbie doesn't get some food soon? Before Arthur falls asleep? Because if he sleeps now he'll scream in the car, then *she* won't sleep, and we haven't got enough milk for later, anyway –'

'Oh, have it your way, let's all go home, let's all shoot ourselves, why do we bloody bother!'

'You are the most unreasonable, selfish pig I have ever –'

But let us pass from these painful scenes. Gathered from a range of enterprising parents, here are some useful observations:

Car travel

Music cassettes help enormously, for all ages from birth onwards. So do toys (dangling from the rear grab-handles above the doors, so that they can't drop them and howl for their return). Best of all, I fear, seems to be an adult in the back. I have a friend who lost his licence for a year and suddenly realized, as his wife smiled a secret little smile, that the magistrate had passed the most appalling sentence possible. He might as well have put on the black cap and said, 'For twelve months you will sit in the back of your car and amuse your two youngest children.' *Twelve months!* Moral: make sure you are the driver.

If you are the sole adult, make sure you install one of those extra rear-view mirrors (they stick on with suction discs to the windscreen) and adjust it to show the face of your dear little passenger. Twisting round is dangerous, even for a moment, but babies learn astonishingly early that certain sicking-up, choking, gagging and teeth-grinding sound-effects will cause the driver to pay them some quick attention for a change (my son did a convincing, and entirely deliberate, death-rattle at 20 months old, starting up every time I stopped singing 'Ukelele Lady' to concentrate on the traffic).

Boating

The very worst age to take children on any kind of small boat is a nine- to eighteen-month-old. New babies and immobile sitting-up ones are not much problem, so long as they have a caretaker and are not sick. But the mobile, inquisitive creature who only wants to range far and wide on knees or wobbly legs is terrible; sulky when held, lethal on the move, resentful of lifejackets, incapable of handling a tangly safety-harness on a big boat. The breakthrough comes somewhere between eighteen months and two and a half when imagination develops, and it suddenly becomes a thrill to be 'on Daddy's big boat!' or 'on a real boat!' and to wear the right kit. The only hope at the difficult age, if you insist on going afloat, is to provide some absolutely riveting, preferably new toy to play with, down on the floorboards; and to get a stout set of reins. As to lifejackets, they are important, almost essential; but may be impossible to get a child under two and a half to wear. Try them on in the shop; some 'jacket' types are better than others for free movement.

Toddlers get enormous satisfaction out of dragging things along behind the boat on a string. Do not forget the string.

Hiking

I know a couple who walked the Pennine Way with a baby in a rucksack-carrier. The only disadvantage, they said airily, was that the other parent has to carry all the gear for all three of you. Youth hostels proved 'extremely helpful' – several times they rang ahead and managed to arrange the hire of a proper cot. At other times, they rigged a sort of frame round a mattress on the floor, out of bits of rucksack lashed with string. You have to be competent and have a dark, morbid imagination to do this sort of thing safely: remember, rolling mobile babies can strangle or wedge themselves in things.

Camping

The great essential is, say bitterly experienced campers, 'a travel cot with opaque sides – so the baby can't see that you're in the same tent and demand to get up at 5 a.m.'

The same couple also discovered that put on to a li-lo, a toddler creeps around and falls off in its sleep; they changed to foam mattresses. The other disconcerting thing about li-los is that if a child wets the bed, it runs like a river in the grooves right down to the bottom and onto whatever food, kit or fellow-camper you have stowed there.

And 'Never bother with a child-size sleeping bag. An ordinary one with the bottom tucked under the mattress, or even tied up with string to stop them getting too far down, is perfect.'

Events, shows, outdoor activity sports

Here the essential is to survey the ground early for sources of drinks, lavatories, shelter and shade. If you have a car, it may need to be a total life-support system, so bring everything you need. Remember that a small child's day needs a bit of boring tranquillity, so be prepared to lurk in the car

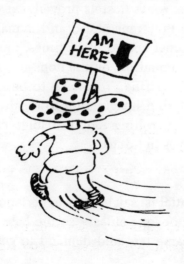

for a while, reading books or listening to music. It helps to put toddlers in very brightly coloured and unusual sunhats so that you can see them if they bolt. Some people use identification bracelets, with the child's surname and address on (never Christian name – makes life too easy for abductors). Personally, I use reins …

Pubs

Some make a positive selling-point out of being child-friendly, with rooms full of soft play equipment and everything shaped like clowns. You may find these insupportable: other people's older children can be a real turn-off for newish parents. As for ordinary pubs in the UK, they are getting better, slowly, although I was once greeted (one step inside a sea-front pub, with a new baby in a sling and a terrible breastfeeding thirst) with the single word, 'Out!' Not: 'Sorry, there isn't a children's room, can you have your drink outside?' but just: 'Out!' Considering all the options, and the fact that I was alone and miles from any other drink, even of water, I just said pleasantly: 'Give me a drink or I'll scream the place down,' and strolled shakily out. He passed me a mug of water in the end, for which I did not pay the requested 10p. However, most pubs with any aspirations at all towards a youthful and family trade provide a room where children are allowed, even if it is a grim corner of the closed dining-room. It is always worth asking, anyway. But more soothing on the whole are:

Teashops

The best piece of equipment we ever had was a clip-on safe seat for a baby, which fixes to any stout table. This saves anyone having the baby on a knee. Later, the Tamsit harness which slips over a chair is quite good (at the stage when they can sit on a chair, but forget where they are at times and topple sideways). Later still, you burst with pride as your eighteen-month-old sits carefully with his orange juice, observing the golden rule: 'Two hands on your mug in a teashop'. The important thing, with both teashops and restaurants, is to find ones where the service is quick. If you have doubts, and two parents, then let one nip in first and do the ordering while the other trundles once more round the block.

Incidentally, it only occurred to me after three gruelling summers of holiday parenthood that there is no strictly biological reason why the mother should always have to stay at the table controlling the children while the father (Man-The-Hunter) queues peacefully at the cafeteria counter.

Swimming
Generally popular with babies from a few months old, with armbands that inflate and warmish water. A brilliant dodge for coaxing toddlers into water they consider too cold is to provide a little blow-pipe for blowing bubbles. Since the only way they can get to blow the bubbles is to be down in the water, it may work wonders. Always has with us.

Parties
The old convention was that children ought never to be exposed to the noise, smoke, booze and decadence of a grown-up party, nor should they be either seen or heard at

a dinner table. This was *very* cramping and restricting to parents.

The *new* convention is that children should *be welcome* everywhere, all the time, play around your feet at intellectual Hampstead dinner parties and feel free to pick up discarded Ecstasy tablets on the floor of trendy clubs. In its way, this is just as bad; it is terrible to be greeted with 'Oh, didn't you bring the baby? We'd love to see her' when you have just exultantly crept out of the house leaving the baby asleep and the sitter doing the ironing. You feel like a heartless mother.

But of course, both the conventions have been happily flouted in their day. Brave mothers in the disapproving 1950s took their carrycots to cocktail parties, and ate dinner occasionally with a toddler on their knee; and conversely, even the most advanced couples of today sometimes firmly suggest to their dinner guests that the dear little two-year-old and the sweet six-month-old baby might be as well off with a babysitter. Because although you can take little babies, asleep, almost anywhere; and although everyone loves an older baby for five minutes at a time, taking them out for the evening does two bad things. It means that *you* stay on duty that bit longer (I have vainly tried to feed, soothe, amuse and relax a couple who had brought their two babies to dinner; in vain – neither of them really seemed to enjoy themselves much for fear of disaster in the corner). And it disrupts the child's routine. A few babies and toddlers can happily be put down to bed in a strange house, picked up at midnight, driven home and decanted into their own bed without protest; but not all of them will do that. A toddler may insist on staying up with the grown-ups. A big baby may cry and cry when he is left, then cry and cry with tiredness and bewilderment downstairs. Things which have helped, in various families, are:

- 'A lambskin baby fleece – used only for sleeping, so wherever you put it down, the baby knows he can sleep safely.'
- 'A bag of familiar books and a familiar mug of juice.'
- 'A very, very long afternoon sleep and a pile of toys in the corner of the dining-room.'
- 'A carrycot – they're out of fashion now, in favour of those clever car-seat-baby-trug things, but they still have their uses. They provide a walled, miniature, private environment in a way a seat can never do; even at two years old our youngest would squeeze into it and be perfectly happy for a few hours anywhere. I suppose it was a womb-substitute.'

One family, very rich, very grand, actually make a point of hiring a babysitter *when they are entertaining at home.* She is there solely to stop the children coming downstairs and disrupting the adults. Another has been known to bring a nanny out to dinner parties, and transform a section of their host's home into a sort of Mary Poppins nursery wing for the night, with only one interruption when the uniformed nanny knocks discreetly on the door to inform Mamma that it is breastfeeding time. But this is Upstairs stuff. Most of us are closer to Downstairs, and the nearest we get is remembering the nifty dodge of taking the baby alarm with us to strange, tall houses.

Hotels

It is worth a long chat with your hotel in advance about exactly what facilities they provide. If you have a travel cot and a big car, it might be easier to take it along than to make some hotel cots safe. Not only are some models actually lethal (the baby's head gets stuck under a bar at the end) but some perfectly safe ones have a knack of rattling horribly whenever the baby moves. I have spent an entire night in a hotel clinging with one hand to the end-post of a metal cot to stop the jingling keeping all three of us awake.

Hotel baths are rarely non-slip, and carrying your own rubber mat around is depressing. One brilliant girl I know takes masking-tape with her, and criss-crosses it on the bottom of the bath for a completely effective non-slip surface which lasts a few days.

'Baby listening' systems operate in some hotels – the system is generally that you leave the 'phone off and they listen every ten minutes or so to see if there is any noise. It is worth reminding the receptionist a few times, and waving a gurgling smiling baby at him or her earlier, in case they forget and don't hear the baby screaming for twenty minutes or more – which may mean, with an older, aware baby, that even after you *do* come it spends the rest of the night too nervous to sleep properly. If you actually leave the hotel, it is essential to get a babysitter. With small babies, I have always rung the local nursing agency and asked for someone; or found a local contact with reliable knowledge of babysitters.

I fear that American hotel chains are better about small children than British ones. There is a hotel tradition in Britain of providing pomp and trimmings without real help or service – plenty of 'sir' and 'madam' and silver-service, but no chance of boiled water at odd hours for bottle-making. American hotels in Britain may look horrible and plastic, but your chance of actual help is considerably greater.

In France, Italy and other warm, Catholic countries the welcome given to babies and small children is so genuine that the British parent almost breaks down and cries, overcome by relief at having escaped from the unwelcoming, disapproving, tight-lipped British world. There is something about a beaming waiter tying a big napkin round your tiny child's neck and murmuring, 'Pommes frites pour m'sieur?' which makes you love and forgive the whole nation, even for its public lavatories.

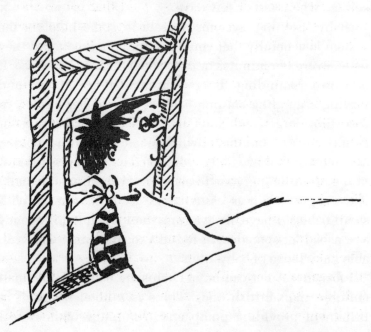

• •

Chapter Eleven

Last Word

For centuries mothers have been helped, worried, supported and oppressed in varying proportions by baby-books. Some of the 'experts' have been pretty unbalanced; a flourishing school of the 1920s held that babies should never be cuddled, but rewarded with a pat on the head or a handshake; even Mrs Sydney Frankenburg, herself a formidable mother, held that nobody should ever point anything out to a toddler, lest he become overstimulated and divert blood to his brain which should be building up his teeth. I am probably unbalanced myself, in some direction or another, although I did write directly from the coalface of motherhood and not from some air-conditioned office up at the pithead. So I would not want the last word. There is no last word, anyway, in this strange world of babies: creatures who are at one moment part of your body, at the next alien, demanding, baffling individuals who take three years to grow to anything like reason (and fifteen more to consolidate it). Any last words in this book will have to come directly from the mothers themselves: the friends whose help, advice and withering criticism have supported this book from the start. I asked them if there was anything they wished they had known at the start of motherhood, or which had proved particularly useful. The last words are theirs:

- 'I wish I had known that two-hourly breastfeeding is perfectly normal, and that after six months it is a waste of time to sterilize everything.'
- '... that how much they eat does not matter. They won't starve, and the more concerned you are with their food, the less they enjoy it.'
- '... that it all goes so quickly. Once school starts, they're gone.'
- '... that you don't actually need a highchair.'
- '... that children are far more tough and resilient than one ever imagines with the first fragile little bundle.'
- '... that they *will* survive if they cry themselves to sleep occasionally.'
- '... that baby-books and mothers-in-law can be a snare.'
- 'What helps? Money and the extended family are the only things that help.'
- 'It helps to forget perfection. If you can get your husband to do anything, whether it's pulling the curtains, putting a nappy on or doing the child's hair, then just say thank you, hold your tongue, and straighten it later if you must. Each of a couple should really be able to cope without too much turmoil if suddenly left on their own.'
- 'It helps not to try and do everything in one day. My granny had a wash day, a baking day, a shopping day etc. She didn't have any machines, but she took her

time and didn't expect too much of herself in one day.'

- 'Oh, if one could only relax! Why else are first children so often anxious and dutiful, while the second-born is a carefree show-off?'

- 'Don't set yourself up to be a martyr or, equally awful, to conduct an exclusive love-affair with your baby. Keep your own life going.'

- 'Have a husband who adores corned beef and baked beans, or cooks. Get out for a walk once a day in all weathers. Put things away. If the house is a shambles, and you see guests arriving, plug in the Hoover and throw a duster somewhere – it looks as if you were about to do something about the mess.'

- 'Rethink all your ideas about everything. Most of them are questionable. Well, mine are.'

- 'Never fight any point unless you have to. Why *can't* she wear her pyjamas all day and clothes all night?'

- 'Realize that *you* are the card your children have drawn. To some extent, they have to come to terms with that. Later on, you come to realize that your children are the cards *you* have drawn, and the same process applies.'

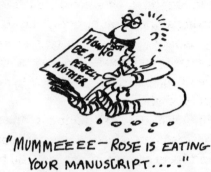

"MUMMEEEE – ROSE IS EATING
YOUR MANUSCRIPT...."

- 'An involved, participating father makes all the difference in the world to every single thing. Work at it.'
- 'Laugh. Cry too, but mainly laugh.'
- 'There are many, many ways of being a good mother. Your way may not be the same as your neighbour's, your sister's or the baby-writer's.'

Index